Prevention of Mental Health Disorders: Principles and Implementation

Editors

ARADHANA BELA SOOD
JIM HUDZIAK

CHILD AND ADOLESCENT PSYCHIATRIC CLINICS OF NORTH AMERICA

www.childpsych.theclinics.com

Consulting Editor
HARSH K. TRIVEDI

April 2016 • Volume 25 • Number 2

ELSEVIER

1600 John F. Kennedy Boulevard ● Suite 1800 ● Philadelphia, Pennsylvania, 19103-2899

http://www.theclinics.com

CHILD AND ADOLESCENT PSYCHIATRIC CLINICS OF NORTH AMERICA Volume 25, Number 2
April 2016 ISSN 1056–4993, ISBN-13: 978-0-323-41746-4

Editor: Lauren Boyle
Developmental Editor: Kristen Helm

Child and Adolescent Psychiatric Clinics of North America (ISSN 1056-4993) is published quarterly by Elsevier Inc., 360 Park Avenue South, New York, NY 10010-1710. Months of issue are January, April, July, and October. Business and Editorial Offices: 1600 John F. Kennedy Boulevard, Suite 1800, Philadelphia, PA 19103-2899. Periodicals postage paid at New York, NY and additional mailing offices. Subscription prices are $310.00 per year (US individuals), $544.00 per year (US institutions), $100.00 per year (US students), $360.00 per year (Canadian individuals), $662.00 per year (Canadian institutions), $200.00 per year (Canadian students), $430.00 per year (international individuals), $662.00 per year (international institutions), and $200.00 per year (international students). International air speed delivery is included in all *Clinics* subscription prices. All prices are subject to change without notice. **POSTMASTER:** Send address changes to *Child and Adolescent Psychiatric Clinics of North America*, Elsevier Health Sciences Division, Subscription Customer Service, 3251 Riverport Lane, Maryland Heights, MO 63043. **Customer Service: 1-800-654-2452 (U.S. and Canada); 314-447-8871 (outside U.S. and Canada). Fax: 314-447-8029. E-mail:** JournalsCustomer Service-usa@elsevier.com **(for print support) or** journalsonlinesupport-usa@elsevier.com **(for online support).**

Reprints. For copies of 100 or more of articles in this publication, please contact the Commercial Reprints Department, Elsevier Inc., 360 Park Avenue South, New York, New York 10010-1710 Tel.: 212-633-3874; Fax: 212-633-3820, E-mail: reprints@elsevier.com.

Child and Adolescent Psychiatric Clinics of North America is covered in *MEDLINE/PubMed (Index Medicus), ISI, SSCI, Research Alert, Social Search, Current Contents,* and *EMBASE/Excerpta Medica.*

Contributors

CONSULTING EDITOR

HARSH K. TRIVEDI, MD, MBA
Executive Director and Chief Medical Officer; Behavioral Health Vice Chair for Clinical Affairs; Associate Professor of Psychiatry, Vanderbilt University School of Medicine, Nashville, Tennessee

CONSULTING EDITOR EMERITUS

ANDRÉS MARTIN, MD, MPH

FOUNDING CONSULTING EDITOR

MELVIN LEWIS, MBBS, FRCPSYCH, DCH

EDITORS

ARADHANA BELA SOOD, MD, MSHA, FAACAP
Professor, Psychiatry and Pediatrics; Senior Professor of Child Mental Health Policy, Virginia Treatment Center for Children, Virginia Commonwealth University, Richmond, Virginia

JIM HUDZIAK, MD
Professor of Psychiatry, Medicine, Pediatrics, and Communication Sciences and Disorders, Director of the Vermont Center for Children, Youth, and Families and The Division of Child Psychiatry, Thomas M. Achenbach Endowed Chair of Developmental Psychopathology, University of Vermont College of Medicine/Fletcher Allen Health Care; Adjunct Professor of Psychiatry (Child), Washington University School of Medicine, St Louis, Missouri; Adjunct Professor in Psychiatry, Geisel School of Medicine at Dartmouth, Burlington, Vermont; Visiting Professor, Erasmus MC, Sophia Children's Hospital, Rotterdam, The Netherlands

AUTHORS

ALEXIS APLASCA, MD
Assistant Professor, Pediatrics and Psychiatry, Children's Hospital of Richmond/Virginia Treatment Center for Children, Virginia Commonwealth University School of Medicine, Richmond, Virginia

STEVEN J. BERKOWITZ, MD
Associate Professor of Clinical Psychiatry, Department of Psychiatry, Perelman School of Medicine, University of Pennsylvania, Philadelphia, Pennsylvania

CHRISTINA BETHELL, PhD, MBA, MPH
Professor, Department of Population, Family and Reproductive Health, Child and Adolescent Health Measurement Initiative, Johns Hopkins Bloomberg School of Public Health, Baltimore, Maryland

JOHN N. CONSTANTINO, MD
Blanche F. Ittleson Professor of Psychiatry and Pediatrics, Division of Child Psychiatry, Department of Psychiatry, Washington University School of Medicine, St Louis, Missouri

TEANIESE LATHAM DAVIS, PhD, MPH
Assistant Professor, Public Health Sciences Institute, Morehouse College, Atlanta, Georgia

RALPH DiCLEMENTE, PhD
Professor, Department of Behavioral Sciences and Health Education, Rollins School of Public Health, Emory University, Atlanta, Georgia

STACY S. DRURY, MD, PhD
Associate Professor, Vice Chair of Research, Department of Psychiatry and Behavioral Sciences, Tulane University, New Orleans, Louisiana

PAUL H. DWORKIN, MD
Professor of Pediatrics; Executive Vice President for Community Child Health, Department of Pediatrics, Office for Community Child Health, *Help Me Grow* National Center, Connecticut Children's Medical Center, University of Connecticut School of Medicine, Hartford, Connecticut

NARANGEREL GOMBOJAV, MD, PhD
Department of Population, Family and Reproductive Health, Child and Adolescent Health Measurement Initiative, Johns Hopkins Bloomberg School of Public Health, Baltimore, Maryland

JIM HUDZIAK, MD
Professor of Psychiatry, Medicine, Pediatrics, and Communication Sciences and Disorders, Director of the Vermont Center for Children, Youth, and Families and The Division of Child Psychiatry, Thomas M. Achenbach Endowed Chair of Developmental Psychopathology, University of Vermont College of Medicine/Fletcher Allen Health Care; Adjunct Professor of Psychiatry (Child), Washington University School of Medicine, St Louis, Missouri; Adjunct Professor in Psychiatry, Geisel School of Medicine at Dartmouth, Burlington, Vermont; Visiting Professor, Erasmus MC, Sophia Children's Hospital, Rotterdam, The Netherlands

MASHA Y. IVANOVA, PhD
Assistant Professor of Psychiatry and Psychology, University of Vermont College of Medicine and University of Vermont Medical Center, Burlington, Vermont

SEAN R. LeNOUE, MD
Fellow, Child and Adolescent Psychiatry, Children's Hospital Colorado, University of Colorado Hospital, University of Colorado School of Medicine, Aurora, Colorado; Chief Resident, Department of Psychiatry, Denver Health Medical Center, Denver, Colorado

TAMAR MENDELSON, PhD
Associate Professor, Department of Mental Health, Johns Hopkins Bloomberg School of Public Health, Baltimore, Maryland

KERRY O'LOUGHLIN, BA
Department of Psychological Science, The University of Vermont, Burlington, Vermont

DUSTIN PARDINI, PhD
Associate Professor, School of Criminology and Criminal Justice, Arizona State University, Phoenix, Arizona

SARA PAWLOWSKI, MD
Fellow, Child and Adolescent Psychiatry, University of Vermont Medical Center, Burlington, Vermont

DAVID C. RETTEW, MD
Associate Professor of Psychiatry and Pediatrics; Training Director, Child and Adolescent Psychiatry Fellowship; Director, Pediatric Psychiatry Clinic, University of Vermont College of Medicine, Burlington, Vermont

PAULA D. RIGGS, MD
Professor and Director, Division of Substance Dependence, Department of Psychiatry, University of Colorado School of Medicine, Aurora, Colorado

LAURA SCARAMELLA, PhD
Professor and Chair, Department of Psychology, The University of New Orleans, New Orleans, Louisiana

LEIGH SMALL, PhD, RN, CPNP-PC, FNAP, FAANP, FAAN
Associate Professor, Department Chair, Family and Community Health Nursing Department, Virginia Commonwealth University School of Nursing, Richmond, Virginia

MICHELE SOLLOWAY, PhD, MPA, RPP
Assistant Scientist, Department of Population, Family and Roproductive Health, Child and Adolescent Health Measurement Initiative, Johns Hopkins Bloomberg School of Public Health, Baltimore, Maryland

ARADHANA BELA SOOD, MD, MSHA, FAACAP
Professor, Psychiatry and Pediatrics; Senior Professor of Child Mental Health Policy, Virginia Treatment Center for Children, Virginia Commonwealth University, Richmond, Virginia

S. DARIUS TANDON, PhD
Associate Professor, Department of Medical Social Sciences and Institute for Public Health and Medicine, Northwestern University Feinberg School of Medicine, Chicago, Illinois

HOLLY C. WILCOX, PhD
Department of Psychiatry and Behavioral Sciences, Johns Hopkins University School of Medicine; Department of Mental Health, Johns Hopkins Bloomberg School of Public Health, Baltimore, Maryland

LAWRENCE WISSOW, MD, PhD
Professor, Department of Health, Behavior and Society, Johns Hopkins Bloomberg School of Public Health, Baltimore, Maryland

PETER A. WYMAN, PhD
Department of Psychiatry, University of Rochester School of Medicine and Dentistry, University of Rochester Medical Center, Rochester, New York

ROSS A. YAPLE, MD
Assistant Professor of Psychiatry, Division of Child and Adolescent Psychiatry, Virginia Treatment Center for Children, Children's Hospital of Richmond, Virginia Commonwealth University Health System, Richmond, Virginia

CHARLES H. ZEANAH, MD
Sellars-Polchow Professor of Psychiatry, Department of Psychiatry and Behavioral Sciences, Tulane University, New Orleans, Louisiana

Contents

> US children with emotional, mental, or behavioral conditions (EMB) have disproportionate exposure to adverse childhood experiences (ACEs). There are theoretic and empirical explanations for early and lifelong physical, mental, emotional, educational, and social impacts of the resultant trauma and chronic stress. Using mindfulness-based, mind–body approaches (MBMB) may strengthen families and promote child resilience and success. This article examines associations between EMB, ACEs, and protective factors, such as child resilience, parental coping/stress, and parent–child engagement. Findings encourage family-centered and mindfulness-based approaches to address social and emotional trauma and potentially interrupt cycles of ACEs and prevalence of EMB.

> Child maltreatment is one of the most deleterious known influences on the mental health and development of children. This article briefly reviews a complement of methods that are ready to incorporate into child and adolescent psychiatric practice, by having been validated either with respect to the prevention of child maltreatment or with respect to adverse outcomes associated with maltreatment (and primarily focused on enhancing the caregiving environment); they are feasible for integration into clinical decision making, and most importantly, can be included in the training of the next generation of clinicians.

> All health is tied to emotional and behavioral health. To improve population health, we need innovative approaches to healthcare that target emotional and behavioral health. The Vermont Family Based Approach (VFBA) is a healthcare paradigm that aims to improve population health by improving emotional and behavioral health. Because the family is a powerful health-promoting social institution, the VFBA also aims to shift the delivery of healthcare to the family level. This article introduces the VFBA, and presents the main empirical findings that informed the approach in the context of the early childhood period.

to increase detection of bullying are indicated, especially among youth presenting with school phobia, depression, anxiety, and declining school performance. Several antibullying efforts have been developed and promoted at the school and community level. Research indicates that many of these programs are effective and share some common elements that can help reduce the prevalence and impact of bullying.

The causes of youth violence are multifactorial and include biological, individual, familial, social, and economic factors. The influence of parents, family members, and important adults can shape the beliefs of the child toward violence in a significant manner. However, the influence of school and the neighborhood also have an important role in attitudes and behaviors of children toward violence. The complexity of factors related to violence requires a comprehensive public health approach. This article focuses on evidence-based models of intervention to reduce violence while emphasizing collective impact as a guiding principle.

Juvenile crime is a serious public health problem that results in significant emotional and financial costs for victims and society. Using etiologic models as a guide, multiple interventions have been developed to target risk factors thought to perpetuate the emergence and persistence of delinquent behavior. Evidence suggests that the most effective interventions tend to have well-defined treatment protocols, focus on therapeutic approaches as opposed to external control techniques, and use multimodal cognitive-behavioral treatment strategies. Moving forward, there is a need to develop effective policies and procedures that promote the widespread adoption of evidence-based delinquency prevention practices across multiple settings.

Prevalence rates of childhood obesity have risen steeply over the last 3 decades. Given the increased national focus, the frequency of this clinical problem, and the multiple mental health factors that coexist with it, make obesity a public health concern. The complex relationships between mental health and obesity serve to potentiate the severity and interdependency of each. The purpose of this review is to create a contextual connection for the 2 conditions as outlined by the research literature and consider treatment options that affect both health problems.

Human immunodeficiency virus (HIV) is the virus that causes AIDS. Surveillance data from 2012 indicate an estimated 1.2 million people aged

Lastly, this article also outlines emerging youth development programs. The model and emerging programs reviewed have resulted in myriad positive outcomes.

CHILD AND ADOLESCENT PSYCHIATRIC CLINICS

AACAP Members: Please go to www.jaacap.org for information on access to the Child and Adolescent Psychiatric Clinics. *Resident* Members of AACAP: Special access information is available at www.childpsych.theclinics.com.

THE CLINICS ARE AVAILABLE ONLINE!
Access your subscription at:
www.theclinics.com

Preface

Prevention of Mental Health Disorders: Principles and Implementation

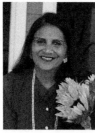 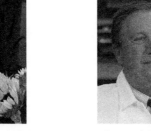

Aradhana Bela Sood, MD, MSHA, FAACAP   Jim Hudziak, MD
Editors

Health care in the United States was once considered to be the best in the world; however, this is no longer true. When measured in terms of life expectancy and health care costs, the United States ranks at the bottom of developed countries. While it is true that the United States continues to lead the world in innovations, we have made little progress in advancing treatments in the common medical problems that lead to premature death and account for the vast majority of health care costs in our country.[1] As concluded by the Robert Wood Johnson Foundation report, "Time to act: investing in the health of our children and communities," it is time for our country to take a more "health focused approach to medical care in our country." To put it simply, it is time to develop new strategies to help the healthy stay well, prevent those at risk for developing illness from becoming ill, and to innovate new ways to help those who are already ill. Overwhelming evidence points to prevention of illness in high-risk individuals as a logical step to reduce later health care problems and stem the rising cost of treatment.[2] Moreover, there is emerging evidence that promoting health may be even more powerful than focused prevention approaches. Despite this compelling argument, there is little funding allocated to health-promotion and illness-prevention programs. However, the gradual recognition that prevention is essential to the future of health and wellness by policymakers in national health care innovation think tanks is slowly creating a momentum to establish the evidence base for these programs. What holds promise is if policy at a legislative level could create a *shared* agenda of advocacy for intervention and prevention efforts rather than dichotomizing the two. This could lead to a fiscally supported prevention strategy. A public health approach where health and wellness

Child Adolesc Psychiatric Clin N Am 25 (2016) xiii–xv
http://dx.doi.org/10.1016/j.chc.2016.01.001
1056-4993/16/$ – see front matter © 2016 Published by Elsevier Inc.

childpsych.theclinics.com

are embedded and incorporated into traditional tertiary care holds promise to positively impact collective population health.

Just how to promote health and prevent illness is no longer such a mystery. Those of us who have contributed to this issue of the *Child and Adolescent Psychiatric Clinics of North America* share a core belief in the following central thesis: "All health emerges from emotional-behavioral health." Why an individual abuses alcohol, drugs, his or her body, or family members is an emotional behavioral act. Similarly, why an individual would engage in health-promoting activities, such as daily exercise, mindfulness, healthy nutrition, making music, mentoring others, and parenting with compassion, is also an emotional behavioral act. It is our contention that all children and families will benefit from the knowledge, skills, and attitudes that will allow them to promote healthy behavior and thus lead to the prevention of the development of a wide variety of common illnesses.

This issue of the *Child and Adolescent Psychiatric Clinics of North America* thus focuses on health-promotion and illness-prevention strategies developed by child and adolescent mental health experts. The articles are organized using a universal, selective, and indicated structure consistent with a public health approach that embraces global and focused health-promotion and illness-prevention approaches while acquainting the reader with the evidence that exists to support each approach. We have organized it into four broad areas through health-promotion and illness-prevention strategies for the common correlates of illness: (1) socioemotional development, wellness, and adversity, which forms the foundation of all health; (2) internalizing and externalizing behavioral syndromes, such as depression, suicide, bullying, youth violence, and delinquency; (3) special topics such as obesity and HIV, and; (4) a model illustrating how prevention has impacted policy at a state level followed by an appendix that provides the reader with an annotated compendium of prevention programs around the country that hold promise or are supported by evidence.

We hope this issue whets the reader's appetite to consider how health-promotion and illness-prevention efforts could be incorporated into clinical practice and into school-based programs and how they could inform advocacy efforts, and even more ambitiously, that the material will spur the reader to consider a career in health promotion and preventive child and adolescent mental health.

Aradhana Bela Sood, MD, MSHA, FAACAP
Virginia Treatment Center for Children
Virginia Commonwealth University
515 North 10th Street
Richmond, VA 23298, USA

Jim Hudziak, MD
University of Vermont
College of Medicine/
Fletcher Allen Health Care
Erasmus MC
Sophia Children's Hospital
Rotterdam, The Netherlands

Washington University School
of Medicine
St Louis, MO, USA

Geisel School of Medicine at Dartmouth
UHC Campus
St. Joe's Room 3213
Box 364SJ 3
1 South Prospect
Burlington, VT 05401, USA

E-mail addresses:
bsood@mcvh-vcu.edu (A.B. Sood)
James.Hudziak@uvm.edu (J. Hudziak)

REFERENCES

1. Robert Wood Johnson Foundation Commission. Time to act: Investing in the health of our children and communities. Executive Summary, Recommendations from the Robert Wood Johnson Foundation Commission to Build a Healthier America; 2014.
2. Prevention for a Healthier America: Trust for Americas Health. Investments in disease prevention yield significant savings, stronger communities. Washington, DC: Trust for Americas Health; 2008. Available at. www.healthyamericans.org. Accessed January 30, 2016.

Adverse Childhood Experiences, Resilience and Mindfulness-Based Approaches

Common Denominator Issues for Children with Emotional, Mental, or Behavioral Problems

Christina Bethell, PhD, MBA, MPH[a],*, Narangerel Gombojav, MD, PhD[a],
Michele Solloway, PhD, MPA, RPP[a], Lawrence Wissow, MD, PhD[b]

KEYWORDS

- Child and adolescent mental health • Adverse childhood experiences • Resilience
- Protective factors • Parent stress • Mindfulness

KEY POINTS

- Compared with children with no adverse childhood experiences (ACEs), prevalence of emotional, mental, or behavioral conditions (EMB) is 1.65 to 4.46 times higher across ACEs levels.
- Those without resilience and multiple ACEs have nearly 11 times greater adjusted odds of having an EMB compared with children with resilience and no ACEs.
- With resilience, children with EMB and multiple ACEs have 1.85 times higher rates of school engagement and are 1.32 times less likely to miss 2 or more school weeks.
- Resilience is nearly 2 times greater among children with EMB and multiple ACEs when their parents report less parenting stress and more engagement in their child's life.
- Attenuating effects of child resilience, parental stress management, and engagement suggest promotion of these protective factors. Mindfulness-based, mind–body methods hold promise for doing so.

Funding Source: This study was supported by the Child and Adolescent Health Measurement Initiative (CAHMI) and by a grant from the National Center for Complementary and Alternative Medicine (R21AT004960). Funded by the National Institutes of Health.
Financial Disclosure: The authors have no financial relationships relevant to this article to disclose.
Conflict of Interest: The authors have no conflicts of interest to disclose.
[a] Child and Adolescent Health Measurement Initiative, Department of Population, Family and Reproductive Health, Johns Hopkins Bloomberg School of Public Health, 615 North Wolfe Street, Baltimore, MD 21205, USA; [b] Department of Health, Behavior and Society, Johns Hopkins Bloomberg School of Public Health, 624 North Broadway, Baltimore, MD 21205, USA
* Corresponding author. 915 South Wolfe Street, #247, Baltimore, MD 21231.
E-mail address: cbethell@jhu.edu

Abbreviations	
ACEs	Adverse childhood experiences
ADHD	Attention deficit hyperactivity disorder
CAM	Complementary and alternative medicine
EMB	Emotional, mental, or behavioral conditions
MBMB	Mindfulness-based, mind–body methods
MEPS	Medical Expenditure Panel Survey
NHIS	National Health Interview Survey
NSCH	National Survey of Children's Health

Diagnosing resilience begins with an assessment of exposure to adversity and the impact risk factors have on children's experience of wellbeing.
 —*Michael Unger, Professor, Dalhousie University, Author: We Generation*

Without mindfulness, there is no therapy. All growth occurs because you are in a state of mindfulness. Without mindfulness, there is no growth.
 —*Bessel van der Kolk, Professor of Psychiatry, Boston University. Author: The Body Keeps the Score and Treating Traumatic Stress in Children and Adolescents*

INTRODUCTION

An estimated 19.8% of all US children have a chronic condition requiring more than routine health and related services. This prevalence increases to 31.6% for the nearly one-fourth of US children exposed to 2 or more adverse childhood experiences (ACEs),[1] such as those experiences studied in the widely recognized Centers for Disease Control and Prevention and Kaiser Permanente study of adults exposed to ACEs.[2] Adapted for children and parental report, the National Survey of Children's Health (NSCH) now assesses 9 types of ACEs, including serious economic hardship, witnessing or experiencing violence in the neighborhood, alcohol, substance abuse, domestic violence, mental health problems in the home, parental divorce, loss of parents to death or incarceration, and social rejection through racial and ethnic discrimination. Measured in this way, the NSCH findings confirm those from the Centers for Disease Control and Prevention/Kaiser and other studies revealing a linear, dose–response effect of ACEs across a wide range of health and social impacts. This effect is stable even in the absence of more detailed information about the occurrence, frequency, and severity of any specific event or set of experiences. Exposure to ACEs is 71% for all US children in fair or poor health. Additionally, US children exposed to ACEs are substantially and significantly more likely to repeat a grade in school and lack resilience, such as usually or always being able to stay calm and in control when faced with a challenge.[1]

Reports on the NSCH show that 70% of the 7.9% of US children ages 2 to 17 with attention deficit hyperactivity disorder (ADHD) have been exposed to ACEs. Less is known about ACEs prevalence and impact for US children with any type of emotional, mental, or behavioral condition(s) (EMB). Because common symptoms are shared by children exposed to ACEs and those diagnosed with EMB,[3,4] it is important to understand the prevalence of ACEs exposure among children with EMB and how these phenomena are related, and to assess whether adaptations are needed in approaches to the prevention, diagnosis, or treatment of EMB in children who may also carry the social and emotional trauma and chronic stress that can result from ACEs.

Growing neuroscience, epigenetic, social, developmental, epidemiologic, resilience, and other sciences are coming together to explain observed early and lifelong impacts of childhood social and emotional trauma and chronic stress that can arise from ACEs and perhaps, in turn, evolve into or contribute to EMB.[5–12] Catalyzed by this evolution of scientific understanding, and anchored in recognition of safe, stable, and nurturing relationships as a pillar for child and adult health,[13] ACEs, trauma-informed practices (a popular terminology for responding to ACEs), and intergenerational approaches are a growing focus in clinical, early care, educational, and community contexts, especially for children with EMB, for promoting trauma healing and resilience for the entire family.[14–16]

Integral to many of these approaches to addressing the emotional trauma and chronic stress that can arise with ACEs are mindfulness-based, mind–body methods (MBMB), which now enjoy growing evidence of effectiveness to promote trauma healing, resilience, and self-regulation of stress, emotions, and behavior.[17–22] This evidence has accumulated sufficiently for the American Academy of Pediatrics to have begun to develop what is expected to be a forthcoming policy statement on the use of mind–body methods in clinical practice. Systematic reviews of research on MBMB suggest that these methods can attenuate cognitive, behavioral and emotional symptoms of conditions like anxiety, ADHD, and depression, can decrease physical pain, promote positive health behaviors and social functioning and increase school engagement and attendance. Purposeful moment-by-moment presence and self-awareness of one's breathing, body sensations, emotions, and/ or thoughts in a nonjudgmental manner (eg, mindfulness) is a common, cross-cutting component of most mind–body methods, like biofeedback, guided imagery, yoga, hypnosis, and meditation.

Showing the relevance of MBMB to parents, Whitaker and colleagues[17] assessed ACEs exposure, health outcomes, and mindfulness among adults, showing that among persons reporting 3 or more ACEs, those in the highest quartile of mindfulness had a prevalence of multiple health conditions two-thirds that of those in the lowest quartile. Other studies conclude that regardless of the presence of trauma, youth-based mindfulness-based stress reduction training in primary care and other settings is effective in improving self-regulation of stress, improving mental health symptoms, lowering blood pressure, and improving overall coping.[18–22]

Although research has demonstrated that MBMBs, such as mindfulness, yoga, Tai chi, and other forms of meditative movement can be effective for general well-being and to address a wide variety of symptoms and conditions,[23–25] this paper focuses on the promising application of MBMB to children and youth with EMB, most of whom are also exposed to ACEs and may carry trauma and chronic stress owing to these experiences. Specifically, this paper aims to provide further insights into why children with ACEs may (or may not) also experience EMB with the goal to inform burgeoning efforts to both reduce EMB prevalence and impact as well as interrupt intergenerational cycles of ACEs.[13,14] To begin, we examined associations among prevalence of EMB among US children with varying levels of ACEs and by differences in risk regulating factors hypothesized to ameliorate negative effects of ACEs, which research shows are also potentially malleable using MBMB. These factors include child resilience and factors indicative of the presence of safe, stable and nurturing family relationships, such as parental coping and stress and parent–child engagement. Rates of use of MBMB among children with EMB is estimated along with their total expenditures for conventional medical care, which may point to delayed use of MBMB that could attenuate severity and costs of care for children with EMB.

METHODS
Population and Data

This study used data from the 2011-12 NSCH, the 2007 National Health Interview Survey (NHIS), the NHIS Child Complementary and Alternative Medicine (CAM) Supplement and the 2008 Medical Expenditure Panel Survey (MEPS).[26] The NSCH surveyed a representative sample of children ages 0 to 17 (95,677 children, with approximately 1800 per state). Child-level household surveys were conducted with parents or guardians under the leadership of the Maternal and Child Health Bureau and implemented through the National Center for Health Statistics. Analyses here are limited to children ages 2 to 17 owing to age parameters for questions related to whether a child had an EMB. Further stratification occurred where variables were only available for school-age children (ages 6–17). Data were weighted to represent the population of noninstitutionalized children nationally and in each state.

Data from the 2007 NHIS and 2008 MEPS were used as the most recent available that allow linking data from the NHIS CAM Supplement to the MEPS health care expenditures datasets to develop estimates of mind–body methods among children with emotional, mental, and behavioral problems in the United States. To estimate prevalence of EMB conditions and use of mind–body methods, we linked 5 2007 NHIS data files (Family, Imputed Income, Person, Sample Child, and Child CAM Supplement), resulting in an integrated NHIS data file that included 9417 sampled children. To obtain health care expenditure data for children with EMB and who used mind–body methods, we further linked this integrated NHIS file with the 2008 MEPS Full-Year Consolidated Household File, which included the NHIS sampling frame (Panel 13). The NHIS/MEPS linked file contains 2411 sample children and were weighted to represent the US population of children ages 0 to 17. Weights for the NHIS/MEPS linked file were constructed adjusting the MEPS Panel 13 weights to reflect the NHIS probabilities of selection for subsampling of children and then, as recommended, weights were further adjusted through ranking by age, sex, race/ethnicity, and US geographic region.

Key Measures

As noted, the 2011-12 NSCH ACEs questions are based on those used in the adult Centers for Disease Control and Prevention/Kaiser study, with modifications overseen by a federal Maternal and Child Health Bureau technical expert panel and evaluated through standard survey item testing by the National Center for Health Statistics. The NSCH included 9 ACEs deemed valid for reporting by parents and guardians as outlined.[1] To evaluate associations between EMB and ACEs, an EMB variable was constructed to include whether a child had been told by a doctor or other provider that they currently have ADHD, depression, anxiety, behavior or conduct problems, autism spectrum disorder, developmental delay, or Tourette syndrome. Variables assessing protective factors were also constructed using the NSCH data and included child resilience (defined simply here as usually or always "staying calm and in control when faced with a challenge," for children ages 6–17), engagement in school (a multi-item measure), and missed school days. Variables constructed to assess hypothesized risk regulating associations between EMB, ACEs, and protective family relationship factors included parental coping, parental aggravation and stress owing to parenting, whether a child and parent do well sharing ideas and talking about things that matter, whether a child's parent knows her or his child's friends and participates in child's events and activities, and the mental health status of the child's mother.

For analyses of the NHIS and MEPS data, 6 health conditions or problems asked about in the 2007 NHIS were grouped together to identify children with EMB conditions or problems: (a) parent has ever been told by a health professional that child has ADHD or ADD, (b) parent has been told by a health professional that child experienced depression or phobia/fears in the past 12 months, and/or (c) parent report that child experienced anxiety/stress, incontinence/bed wetting, or insomnia/trouble sleeping in the past 12 months. MBMBs included biofeedback, hypnosis, yoga, Tai chi, Qi gong, meditation, guided imagery, progressive relaxation, deep breathing exercises, support group meeting, and stress management class (like Mindfulness-Based Stress Reduction). Total conventional medical care expenditures estimates were constructed based on standard 2-part models and were adjusted for child's age, sex, race/ethnicity, income, and US region. All variables used in this study have been documented previously, and their properties and coding are presented in publicly available NSCH and NHIS variable codebooks developed by the Child and Adolescent Health Measurement Initiative.[26]

Analytical Methods

Bivariate analyses, rate ratio analyses, χ^2 tests, and t tests were used in addition to multivariate logistic regression models to evaluate variations in prevalence of EMB by a child's ACEs status and to further evaluate these associations by a child's age, household income, resilience, and protective family relationship factors. Similar analyses were conducted to determine the impact of ACEs on school engagement and missed school among children with EMB, and potential mitigating impact when a child had learned and demonstrated resilience. All regression analyses controlled for child age, sex, race/ethnicity, health insurance status/type, and household income (for models not stratified by income). We used SPSS, version 22 (SPSS Inc, Chicago, IL). Unless otherwise noted, all adjusted odds ratios that we report were significant based on their 95% CIs.

RESULTS
Characteristics of US Children with Emotional, Mental, or Behavioral Conditions by Adverse Childhood Experiences Status

Children with EMB are disproportionately older, compared with children generally. This is especially true if they also experience multiple ACEs. Children with EMB are also more likely to be male, regardless of their ACEs status. Independent of their EMB status, children with multiple ACEs are more likely to live in lower income homes and have public insurance; however, those with both ACEs and EMB are especially likely to have public insurance (63.9%). Children without EMB but with multiple ACEs are 1.4 time more likely to be uninsured (**Table 1**).

Prevalence of Emotional, Mental, or Behavioral Conditions by Adverse Childhood Experiences Status, Household Income, and Age of Child

Across levels of ACEs (1, 2–3, $\geq$4), the prevalence of EMB among US children ages 2 to 17 is 1.65 to 4.46 times higher compared with those with no ACEs (**Table 2**). Consistent effects exist across child household income and age groups. Strongest effects are found for younger children (ages 2–5) and those living in households with incomes below 200% of the federal poverty level. Across 4 income categories, the prevalence of EMB is 3.77 to 5.40 greater for children and youth exposed to 4 or more ACEs. Differences in the prevalence of EMB for these children are not significant across income categories ($P = .33$; see **Table 2**). This finding remains for each of the individual conditions included in the EMB measures, with the exception of

Table 1
Demographic and health insurance characteristics among US children age 2-17 with ACEs by emotional, mental, or behavioral health status

Demographic and Health Insurance Characteristics	All US Children, 2-17 y (%)	ACEs, 2-17 y (%)				Children with Emotional, Mental, or Behavioral Problems,[a] 2-17 y (%)		Children with Emotional, Mental, or Behavioral Problems,[a] 2-17 y (%)			Children Without Emotional, Mental, or Behavioral Problems,[a] 2-17 y (%)		
		4 + ACEs	2-3 ACEs	1 ACE	None	Yes	No	No ACEs	1 ACE	≥2 ACEs	No ACEs	1 ACE	≥2 ACEs
All children, 2-17 y	100	7.1	17.6	25.6	49.7	14.0	86.0	29.3	25.0	45.7	53.1	25.7	21.2
Age (y)													
2-5	24.4	11.8	17.1	23.5	29.1	11.2	26.5	13.1	12.5	8.9	30.6	25.3	17.9
6-11	37.3	35.4	37.5	37.4	37.3	39.6	37.0	42.5	37.3	38.9	36.8	37.5	36.2
12-17	38.3	52.8	45.4	39.0	33.6	49.2	36.5	44.5	50.1	52.1	32.6	37.3	45.9
Sex													
Male	51.2	52.4	50.3	51.6	51.3	63.7	49.2	68.3	62.0	61.7	49.8	50.0	47.1
Female	48.8	47.6	49.7	48.4	48.7	36.3	50.8	31.7	38.0	38.3	50.2	50.0	52.9
Race													
Hispanic	23.2	21.8	22.8	26.2	21.8	17.3	24.1	15.8	19.4	17.0	22.4	27.3	24.5
White, non-Hispanic	53.0	50.3	48.1	49.3	57.1	59.2	52.0	66.5	57.1	55.5	56.2	48.1	46.3
Black, non-Hispanic	13.8	16.4	19.5	15.7	10.3	14.8	13.6	10.4	16.4	16.8	10.3	15.5	19.3
Other, non-Hispanic	10.1	11.5	9.6	8.8	10.7	8.8	10.3	7.4	7.1	10.7	11.0	9.0	9.9

Household income (% FPL)												
0–99	21.9	39.1	31.8	26.5	13.6	27.5	21.0	13.8	24.8	38.1	13.6	26.8	32.5
100–199	21.6	28.5	27.1	25.9	16.5	22.9	21.4	13.1	24.7	28.3	16.8	26.1	27.2
200–399	28.5	24.0	27.6	27.5	30.1	26.6	28.8	30.1	28.5	23.4	30.1	27.4	27.7
≥400	28.0	8.4	13.5	20.0	39.8	22.9	28.8	43.0	22.0	10.2	39.5	19.7	12.7
Insurance type													
Public	36.3	63.2	51.7	41.2	24.3	48.4	34.3	27.7	44.7	63.9	24.0	40.7	51.8
Private	57.9	28.4	41.5	52.0	71.2	47.7	59.5	70.1	51.5	31.2	71.3	52.1	40.1
Uninsured	5.8	8.4	6.8	6.8	4.6	3.9	6.1	2.2	3.8	4.9	4.8	7.2	8.1
Insurance adequacy[b]													
Adequate	75.8	74.3	75.0	73.7	77.4	68.8	77.0	68.3	65.6	71.0	78.2	75.0	76.2
Inadequate	24.2	25.7	25.0	26.3	22.6	31.2	23.0	31.7	34.4	29.0	21.8	25.0	23.8

Abbreviations: ACEs, adverse childhood experiences; FPL, federal poverty level.

[a] Defined as children who qualify on the Children with Special Health Care Needs Screener criteria for having emotional, developmental, or behavioral conditions that have lasted or are expected to last for ≥12 months and require treatment or counseling and/or who have had a doctor indicate current presence of ≥1 of 7 emotional, mental, or behavioral conditions asked in the National Survey of Children's Health.

[b] Among currently insured children.

Data from 2011-2012 National Survey of Children's Health.

Table 2
Prevalence of EMB[a] among US children ages 2-17 by ACEs exposure status and household income and age

	EMB Prevalence: All US Children Age 2-17 (%)	EMB Prevalence: Children Age 2-17 with No ACEs (%)	EMB Prevalence: Children Age 2-17 with 1 ACE (%)		EMB Prevalence: Children Age 2-17 with 2-3 ACEs (%)		EMB Prevalence: Children Age 2-17 with ≥4 of 9 ACEs (%)		Ratio of EMB Prevalence	
			%	AOR[b]	%	AOR	%	AOR	No ACEs vs ≥1	No ACEs vs 1, 2-3, or ≥4
All children 2-17 y	14.0	8.3 (ref)	13.7	1.64	21.7	2.62	37.0	5.02	2.39	1.65-4.46
Household income (% FPL)										
0-99	17.6	8.5 (ref)	12.8	1.44	24.0	2.66	40.0	5.21	2.58	1.50-4.70
100-199	14.9	6.6 (ref)	13.1	1.89	23.1	3.34	35.7	5.59	3.04	1.98-5.40
200-399	13.1	8.3 (ref)	14.2	1.69	18.9	2.27	34.8	4.86	2.23	1.71-4.19
≥400	11.5	9.0 (ref)	15.1	1.57	19.2	2.02	33.9	3.67	1.97	1.68-3.77
P value (χ^2)	<.001	.05	.41	—	.03	—	.33	—	—	—
Child age (y)										
2-5	6.4	3.7 (ref)	7.3	1.85	12.6	3.13	23.5	6.59	2.78	1.97-6.35
6-11	14.9	9.5 (ref)	13.7	1.44	23.6	2.69	38.0	5.08	2.16	1.44-4.00
12-17	18.1	11.0 (ref)	17.6	1.75	23.6	2.44	39.4	4.71	2.14	1.60-3.58
P value (χ^2)	.001	.001	.001	—	.001	—	.001	—	—	—

Abbreviations: ACEs, adverse childhood experiences; AOR, adjusted odds ratio; EMB, emotional, mental, or behavioral health conditions; FPL, federal poverty level.

[a] Defined as children who qualify on the Children with Special Health Care Needs Screener criteria for having emotional, developmental, or behavioral conditions that have lasted or are expected to last for ≥12 months and require treatment or counseling and/or who have had a doctor indicate current presence of ≥1 of 7 emotional, mental, or behavioral conditions asked in the National Survey of Children's Health.

[b] Adjusted for age, sex, race/ethnicity, insurance status/type.

Data from 2011-2012 National Survey of Children's Health.

conduct or behavioral problems, which are systematically higher for lower income children with multiple ACEs compared with similar higher income children (data not shown).

Prevalence of Emotional, Mental, or Behavioral Conditions by Adverse Childhood Experiences and Resilience Status

In this study, a single construct of resilience is measured as parental observation of whether their child is usually or always able to stay calm and in control when faced with a challenge. The presence of resilience measured in this minimal way is significantly associated with a lower prevalence of EMB, even for children with no ACEs. On average, the prevalence of EMB is 3.3 times greater when children lack this single aspect of resilience (**Table 3**). Across ACEs status categories (0, 1, ≥2), the prevalence of EMB is 2.64 to 3.35 times greater when children lack this aspect of resilience (**Fig. 1**). Only one-third of US children (33.4%) and 12.8% with EMB are resilient and ACEs free. Although substantial variations exist across income categories, only 28.6% of children with EMB in the highest income category are both resilient and free from ACEs (**Fig. 2**). Compared with the 12.8% of children with EMB who demonstrate resilience and lack ACEs, those without resilience and multiple ACEs are 6.6 times more likely to have an EMB (6.4% vs 42.5%; data not shown). On the contrary, when children with 2 or more ACEs nonetheless demonstrate resilience, they are 2.64 times less likely to have EMB than their peers with 2 or more ACEs who lack resilience (see **Table 3**).

Prevalence of Emotional, Mental, or Behavioral Conditions by School Success Factors, Adverse Childhood Experiences, and Resilience

Children with 2 or more ACEs are 2.39 and 1.91 times more likely to not be engaged in school or missed more than 2 weeks of school, respectively (see **Table 3**). Children with EMB and multiple ACEs have 1.85 times higher rates of school engagement and are 1.32 times less likely to miss 2 or more weeks of school if they demonstrate the aspect of resilience assessed here (**Fig. 3**).

Prevalence of Emotional, Mental, or Behavioral Conditions by Family Protective Factors and Associations with Adverse Childhood Experiences and Resilience

Prevalence of EMB is 1.45 to 3.62 times higher when the following five family-focused protective factors assessed are missing (see **Table 3**): (1) parent-child share ideas and discuss things that matter (rate ratio: 1.92); (2) parent has met most or all of child's friends and usually or always participates in child's events (rate ratio: 1.45); (3) parent manages stress and aggravation with parenting (rate ratio: 3.62); (4) parent copes well with parenting (rate ratio: 1.92); and/or (5) mother's mental health is excellent or very good (rate ratio: 1.82). These variations are somewhat attenuated when children have also been exposed to 2 or more ACEs (1.42–2.64 across the 5 factors), such that those with multiple ACEs are more likely to have EMB, regardless of these factors. Among family protective factors assessed, parental stress and aggravation has the biggest effect on prevalence of EMB for all children, as well as for those with multiple ACEs. For children with multiple ACEs, the effect of having parents who have met all or most of the child's friends and usually or always attend their events is somewhat stronger.

Across all 5 family-focused protective factors, children with EMB are 1.23 to 1.44 times less likely to live in homes where the 5 family-focused protective factors exist compared with children without EMB. Similarly, children with EMB and multiple ACEs are also 1.44 to 2.08 less likely to live in such homes (see **Table 3**). Conversely,

Table 3
Prevalence of EMB[a] among children (2–17 or 6–17 depending on variable) by child resilience and protective factors status: by EMB and among EMB with 2 or more adverse childhood experiences (ACEs: 70.7% EMB have 1 + ACEs)

	EMB Prevalence and Rate Ratios (Children with Negative vs Positive Result on Protective Factor)[b]					Distribution of Children with Protective Factors: by EMB and ACEs Status (Age 2–17 or 6–17 Depending Upon Protective Factor Variable)		
	EMB Prevalence: All Children (%)	EMB RR[c]	EMB Prevalence: Children with ≥2 ACEs (%)	EMB RR[c]	Children with EMB (%)	Children without EMB (%)	Children with EMB and ≥2 ACEs (%)	All Children (%)
Child demonstrates resilience (usually or always stays calm and in control when faced with a challenge; age 6–17)								
Yes	9.1	3.30	16.1	2.64	35.8	70.4	31.3	64.7
No	30.0		42.5		64.2	29.6	68.7	35.3
Parent and child share ideas and talk about things that matter (very well; age 6–17)								
Yes	13.0	1.92	23.4	1.56	55.3	73.3	52.7	70.4
No	24.9		36.6		44.7	26.7	47.3	29.6
Parent has met most/all child's friends and attends most/all of child's events (age 6–17)								
Yes	13.7	1.45	23.1	1.55	48.4	59.7	41.3	57.9
No	19.8		35.9		51.6	40.3	58.7	42.1
Parent is usually or always stressed with parenting or aggravated with child (age 2–17)								
Yes	38.7	3.62	53.3	2.64	32.9	8.5	36.4	11.9
No	10.7		20.2		67.1	91.5	63.6	88.1
Parent reports coping very well with parenting (age 2–17)								
Yes	10.2	1.92	20.6	1.52	42.6	61.6	37.7	59.0
No	19.6		31.3		57.4	38.4	62.3	41.0

			RR			RR			
Mother's mental health excellent/very good (age 2-17)									
Yes	10.9	1.82	21.3	57.3	1.42	72.9	43.7	70.8
No	19.8		30.2	42.7		27.1	56.3	29.2
Child is usually/always engaged in school (age 6-17)									
Yes	11.3	3.35	19.5	55.0	2.39	85.4	46.8	80.4
No	37.9		46.5	45.0		14.6	53.2	19.6
Child missed ≥2 weeks of school/year (age 6-17)									
Yes	38.6	2.59	48.5	14.5	1.91	4.5	18.8	6.2
No	14.9		25.4	85.5		95.5	81.2	93.8

Abbreviations: ACEs, adverse childhood experiences; EMB, emotional, mental, or behavioral health conditions; FPL, federal poverty level; RR, rate ratio.
[a] Defined as children who qualify on the Children with Special Health Care Needs Screener criteria for EMB conditions or current diagnosis of 7 emotional, mental, or behavioral conditions asked in the National Survey of Children's Health.
[b] All EMB prevalence rate differences for each factor are statistically significant at $P \leq 05$.
[c] RR between those with or without the positive valence of the protective factor.
Data from 2011-2012 National Survey of Children's Health.

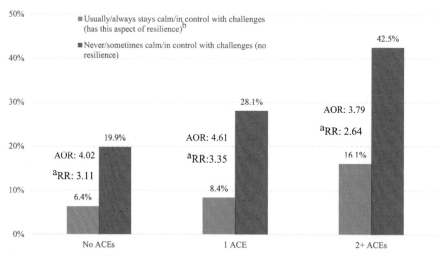

Fig. 1. Prevalence of emotional, mental, or behavioral conditions (EMB) by adverse childhood experiences (ACEs) exposure and resilience status (all US children ages 6–17). [a] All rate ratios (RRs) are statistically significant at $P \leq .05$ and using multivariate logistic regression with adjustment for age, sex, race/ethnicity, household income, and insurance status/type. [b] Reference category for multivariate logistic regression models. AOR, adjusted odds ratio. (*Data from* 2011-2012 National Survey of Children's Health.)

when children with EMB and multiple ACEs live in homes with at least 1 family-focused protective factor, they are 1.27 to 2.05 times more likely to demonstrate resilience. These effects are greatest for children in homes where the parent and child share ideas and discuss things that really matter (**Fig. 4**).

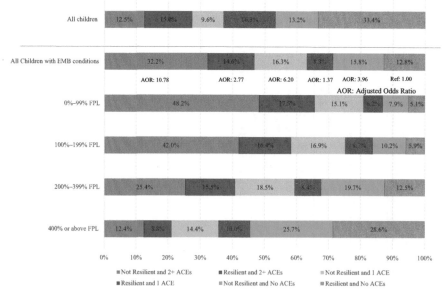

Fig. 2. Distribution of all school age children (6–17) and children with emotional, mental, or behavioral conditions (EMBs): by resilience, adverse childhood experiences (ACEs) status and income (federal poverty level [FPL]). (*Data from* 2011-2012 National Survey of Children's Health.)

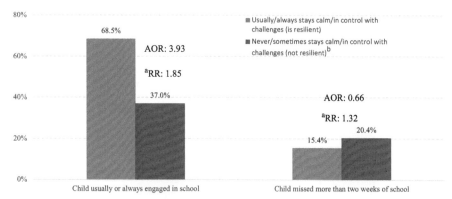

Fig. 3. Prevalence of school success factors among US children age 6 to 17 with emotional, mental or behavioral conditions (EMB) and 2 or more adverse childhood experiences exposures (ACEs) by resilience status. [a] RR, rate ratio. All RRs statistically significant at $P \le .05$ and using multivariate logistic regression with adjustment for age, sex, race/ethnicity, household income, and insurance status/type, [b] Reference category for multivariate logistic regression models. AOR, adjusted odds ratio. (*Data from* 2011-2012 National Survey of Children's Health.)

Use of Risk Regulating Mindfulness-Based, Mind–Body Approaches, and Medical Expenditures

About 5% of US children age 2 to 17 have parents who reported their child has used the MBMB assessed in the NHIS-CAM Supplement. This increases to 14% for children with EMB and to 14.9% for children with ADD/ADHD (**Fig. 5**). Those with any type of EMB who use MBMB used more conventional medical care for their conditions and have 1.82 times higher adjusted total conventional medical expenditures compared with those who did not use MBMB. This effect is similar for children with

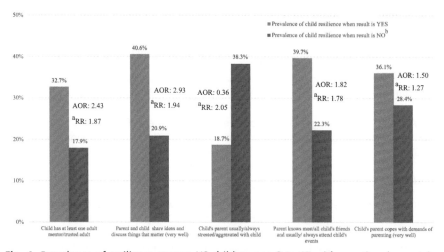

Fig. 4. Prevalence of resilience among US children age 2 to 17 with emotional, mental or behavioral conditions (EMB) and 2 or more adverse childhood experiences (ACEs) exposures by key protective factors. [a] RR, rate ratio. All rate ratios statistically significant at $P \le .05$ and using multivariate logistic regression with adjustment for age, sex, race/ethnicity, household income and insurance status/type. [b] Reference category for multivariate logistic regression models. AOR, adjusted odds ratio. (*Data from* 2011-2012 National Survey of Children's Health.)

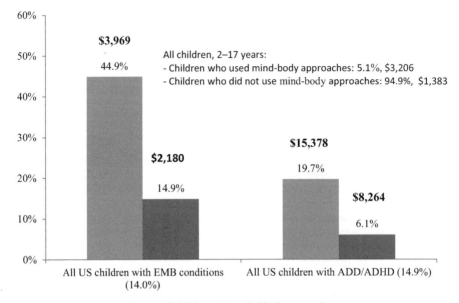

Fig. 5. Use of mind–body approaches and mean of total conventional medical care expenditures for US children age 2 to 17: all children, those with emotional, mental or behavioral conditions (EMB) and those with attention deficit disorder (ADD)/attention deficit hyperactivity disorder (ADHD). RR, rate ratio. EMB conditions include (a) parent has ever been told by a health professional that child has ADHD or ADD, (b) parent told by a health professional that child experienced depression or phobia/fears in the past 12 months, and/or (c) parent reports that child experienced anxiety/stress, incontinence/bed wetting, or insomnia/trouble sleeping in the past 12 months. Mind–body approaches include biofeedback, hypnosis, yoga, tai chi, qi gong, meditation, guided imagery, progressive relaxation, deep breathing exercises, support group meeting, and stress management class/mindfulness-based stress reduction. Expenditures estimated by 2 part-model adjusting for child's age, sex, race/ethnicity, income, and US region child lives in. Percent estimates and estimated mean of total health care expenditures among mind–body users and nonusers statistically significant at $P \leq .05$. (*Data from* 2007 NHIS and NHIS-Child CAM Supplement and 2008 MEPS.)

ADD/ADHD (1.86 times greater adjusted expenditures) and for all children generally (2.32 times greater adjusted expenditures). These differences are significant (see **Fig. 5**).

DISCUSSION

The findings presented herein are the first showing hypothesized associations among EMB, ACEs, resilience, and family protective factors in a population-based sample of US children and youth. In this way, results are critical to confirm more narrowly focused studies[27–29] and are useful to guide rapidly evolving efforts underway nationally to prevent and decrease the impact of EMB and ACEs and promote positive health. This includes the many efforts taking place to integrate primary care and mental and behavioral health services and in educational and other community based settings.[14,16]

The co-occurring nature of EMB, ACEs, and school success factors, and the mediating effects of resilience, parental stress, parent–child engagement, and other family-focused protective factors are likely not surprising to many clinicians and child health leaders. The population-based findings presented here may simply confirm current understanding. Findings also raise questions about the directionality of observed effects. Specifically, because ACEs are largely a function of failures in the safety, stability, and nurturing properties of the child's relationships and environment, by their nature, ACEs challenge a child's capacity to manage stress and build resilience. In this way, lower rates of resilience and protective factors among children with ACEs are not surprising.

What is more revealing here is the relative effect of building a child's resilience and family protective factors to both attenuate the impact of ACEs that have already occurred and associations between these factors and prevalence of EMB, regardless of ACEs status. The cross-cutting attenuating effects of child resilience, parental stress management, and engagement found here suggest the importance of population-based promotion of these protective factors overall and especially for children already exposed to ACEs. MBMB methods hold promise for doing so, yet are used infrequently. When children with EMB do use MBMB, findings suggest they do so after extensive use of conventional medical care approaches. This is indicated by the higher use and costs of medical care expenditures for these children. This suggests that parents turn to MBMB only after their child's condition becomes more severe and they have sought help across a range of health care providers and pharmaceutical treatments.

Although more research is required, these findings hold promise for potentially decreasing health care costs for children and their families, especially those with EMB and exposure to ACEs. Given growing evidence on the effectiveness of MBMB to attenuate symptoms associated with many types of EMB (ADHD, depression, anxiety, conduct disorders), findings from this study suggest a delayed and underuse of MBMB approaches for children.

Findings from this study emphasize the importance of resilience and the quality of the family relationships implicated in a child's ACEs status. In this way, findings support attention to the ACEs status of parents and their own capacities to manage stress and heal from the trauma and chronic stress that can accumulate when exposed to ACEs. Findings may also lead to rethinking the sufficiency and appropriateness of predominant EMB treatment norms, such as the widespread use of pharmaceutical-based treatment plans (eg, 68% of children with ADHD currently take medications)[27] and consider use of mindfulness and other mind-body–based methods in conjunction with more comprehensive clinical approaches that address trauma.

Common, so-called trauma-informed efforts specifically target the prevention and reduction of impacts from ACEs and the chronic stress and trauma that can result and impact health early and across the lifespan. Such approaches are defined, recommended, and supported by the federal Substance Abuse and Mental Health Administration,[30] the federal Centers for Medicare and Medicaid Services,[31] the Administration for Children and Families,[11] and, more recently, by the American Academy of Pediatrics. In particular, although not as yet addressed by many pediatric providers,[32] ACEs are a growing consideration among pediatric clinicians who increasingly share goals to advance resilience and social and emotional well-being of children and youth. We suggest 3 reasons for this: (1) similarities in symptoms of many EMB diagnoses and those associated with exposure to ACEs, (2) the many undiagnosed children with untreated symptoms related to ACEs exposure, and (3) new possibilities for prevention, healing, and treatment introduced by growing neuroscience, epigenetic, resilience, positive health, and mindfulness and mind-body–related research.

A primary limitation of this study is the cross-sectional nature of the NSCH data. Unfortunately, the United States does not have a longitudinal population-based study that includes information on EMB, ACEs, and other variables evaluated herein. Such data, including integration with medical and other services and costs of care and biologic and other environmental measurements, are needed to document causal effects and better understand variations in outcomes between and within risk subgroups. In the absence of a national longitudinal study that includes such data, follow-back surveys among cohorts of children included in the 2011-12 NSCH hold promise, as does the integration of ACEs and protective factors data in existing longitudinal cohort studies. Additional limitations exist to the extent that NSCH items/measures used here lack sensitivity, specificity, or comprehensiveness for the concepts assessed. Generally, surveys such as the NSCH are biased in the direction of positive reporting, suggesting that with improvement the effects observed here likely show even more marked effects of ACEs and lack of resilience and family protective factors.

SUMMARY

Based on a recent United Nations report, the US ranks 26th out of 29 countries in child well-being.[33] We also lag in educational and health care system promotion of resilience and social and emotional skills especially impacted by ACEs and highlighted as critical to health of society and the world in the International Organization for Economic Co-Operation and Development.[34] Many would attribute these embarrassing results to failures to strengthen families and communities and the proactive promotion of social and emotional skills of children and all people; skills especially impacted by ACEs and effecting generations of children if not addressed.[35]

As the call for the transformation of the US health care system grows, clinicians, policymakers, educators, and system leaders are challenged to catalyze and foster a model of health care focused on the proactive pursuit of whole person, whole family, and whole population health and well-being. This paper further confirms the importance of addressing the growing prevalence of EMB, ACEs, and risk regulating protective factors that are potentially malleable using MBMB, such as child resilience, parental coping and stress, and parent–child engagement. Rates of use of MBMB among children with EMB in the United States suggest delayed and underuse of these promising methods.[36–38] Findings support integrated, family-centered, and mindfulness-based trauma-informed approaches to address social and emotional trauma and interrupt intergenerational cycles of ACEs and their contribution to EMB among children and youth.

REFERENCES

1. Bethell CD, Newacheck P, Hawes E, et al. Adverse childhood experiences: assessing the impact on health and school. Engagement and the mitigating role of resilience. Health Aff 2014;33(12):2106–15.
2. Injury Prevention & Control: Division of Violence Prevention. Adverse childhood experiences. Centers for Disease Control and Prevention. Available at: www.cdc.gov/violenceprevention/acestudy/. Accessed October 10, 2015.
3. Rahim M. Developmental trauma disorder: an attachment-based perspective. Clin Child Psychol Psychiatry 2014;19(4):548–60.
4. Schmid M, Petermann F, Fegert JM. Developmental trauma disorder: pros and cons of including formal criteria in the psychiatric diagnostic systems. BMC Psychiatry 2013;13:3.

5. Garner AS, Forkey H, Szilagyi M. Translating developmental science to address childhood adversity. Acad Pediatr 2015;15(5):493–502.

6. McEwen BS, Gianaros PJ. Central role of the brain in stress and adaptation: links to socioeconomic status, health, and disease. Ann N Y Acad Sci 2010;1186(1): 190–222. Blackwell Publishing Inc.

7. Institute of Medicine and National Research Council. Preventing mental, emotional, and behavioral disorders among young people: progress and possibilities. Washington, DC: The National Academies Press; 2009.

8. Shonkoff JP, Boyce W, McEwen BS. Neuroscience, molecular biology, and the childhood roots of health disparities: building a new framework for health promotion and disease prevention. JAMA 2009;301(21):2252–9.

9. Van der Kolk B. The body keeps the score: brain, mind, and body in the healing of trauma. New York: Penguin Books; 2014.

10. Zannas AS, West AE. Epigenetics and the regulation of stress vulnerability and resilience. Neuroscience 2014;264:157–70.

11. Hamoudi A, Murray DW, Sorensen L, et al. Self-regulation and toxic stress: a review of ecological, biological, and developmental studies of self-regulation and stress. OPRE Report # 2015-30. Washington, DC: Office of Planning, Research and Evaluation, Administration for Children and Families, US Department of Health and Human Services; 2015.

12. Ungar M, Ghazinour M, Richter J. Annual research review: what is resilience within the social ecology of human development? J Child Psychol Psychiatry 2013;54:348–66.

13. Sege R, Linkenbach J. Essentials for childhood: promoting healthy outcomes from positive experiences. Pediatrics 2014;133(6):e1489–91.

14. Flynn AB, Fothergill KE, Wilcox HC, et al. Primary care interventions to prevent or treat traumatic stress in childhood: a systematic review. Acad Pediatr 2015;15(5):480–92.

15. Fraser JG, Lloyd SW, Murphy RA, et al. Child exposure to trauma: comparative effectiveness of interventions addressing maltreatment. Comparative Effectiveness Review No 89. (Prepared by the RTIUNC Evidence-based Practice Center under Contract No. 290-2007-10056-I.) AHRQ Publication No. 13-EHC002-EF. Rockville (MD): Agency for Healthcare Research and Quality; 2013.

16. Wissow LS, Brown J, Fothergill KE, et al. Universal mental health screening in pediatric primary care: a systematic review. J Am Acad Child Psychiatry 2013; 52(11):1134–47.e23.

17. Whitaker RC, Dearth-Wesley T, Gooze RA, et al. Adverse childhood experiences, dispositional mindfulness, and adult health. Prev Med 2014;67:147–53.

18. Black DS. Mindfulness training for children and adolescents: a state-of-the-science review. In: Brown KW, Creswell JD, Ryan RM, editors. Handbook of mindfulness: theory, research, and practice. New York: Guilford Press; 2015. p. 283–310.

19. Felver JC, Celis-de Hoyos CE, Tezanos K, et al. A systematic review of mindfulness-based interventions for youth in school settings. Mindfulness 2015. [Epub ahead of print].

20. Kallapiran K, Koo S, Kirubakaran R, et al. Effectiveness of mindfulness in improving mental health symptoms of children and adolescents: a meta-analysis. Child Adolesc Ment Health 2015;20(4):182–94.

21. Takimoto-Ohnishi E, Ohnishi J, Murakami K. Mind–body medicine: effect of the mind on gene expression. Personalized Medicine Universe 2012;1(1):2–6.

22. Harnett PS, Dawe S. Review: The contribution of mindfulness-based therapies for children and families and proposed conceptual integration. Child and Adolescent Mental Health 2012;17(4):195–208.

23. Hempel S, Taylor SL, Marshall NJ, et al. Evidence map of mindfulness. Project #05–226. Washington, DC: Department of Veterans Affairs (US); 2014.
24. Coeytaux RR, McDuffie J, Goode A, et al. Evidence map of yoga for high-impact conditions affecting veterans. Project #09–010. Washington, DC: Department of Veterans Affairs (US); 2014.
25. Hempel S, Taylor SL, Solloway M, et al. Evidence map of Tai Chi. Project #05–226. Washington, DC: Department of Veterans Affairs (US); 2014.
26. Child and Adolescent Health Measurement Initiative, Data Resource Center for Child and Adolescent Health. Learn about the surveys. Available at: www.child-healthdata.org. Accessed September 17, 2015.
27. Howie LD, Pastor PN, Lukacs SL. Use of medication prescribed for emotional or behavioral difficulties among children aged 6–17 years in the United States, 2011–2012. NCHS data brief, no 148. Hyattsville (MD): National Center for Health Statistics; 2014.
28. Kerker BD, Zhang J, Nadeem E, et al. Adverse childhood experiences and mental health, chronic medical conditions, and development in young children. Acad Pediatr 2015;15(5):510–7.
29. Fuller-Thomson E, Lewis DA. The relationship between early adversities and attention-deficit/hyperactivity disorder. Child Abuse Negl 2015;47:94–101.
30. Substance Abuse and Mental Health Services Administration. Adverse childhood experiences. [Internet]. Rockville (MD): SAMHSA. Available at: http://captus.samhsa.gov/prevention-practice/targeted-prevention/adverse-childhood-experiences/1. Accessed October 31, 2014.
31. Sheldon GH, Tavenner M, Hyde PS. Letter to state directors [Internet]. Washington, DC: Department of Health and Services; 2013. Available at: http://medicaid.gov/Federal-Policy-Guidance/Downloads/SMD-13-07-11.pdf. Accessed October 31, 2014.
32. Kerker BD, Storfer-Isser A, Szilagyi M, et al. Do pediatricians ask about adverse childhood experiences in pediatric primary care? Acad Pediatr 2015. [Epub ahead of print].
33. UNICEF Office of Research. Child well-being in rich countries: a comparative overview, innocenti report card 11. Florence (Italy): UNICEF Office of Research; 2013. Available at: www.unicef-irc.org/publications/pdf/rc11_eng.pdf. Accessed October 10, 2015.
34. Office of Economic Cooperation and Development (OECD). Skills for social progress: the power of social and emotional skills, OECD skills studies. Paris (France): OECD Publishing; 2015.
35. Schor EL, Menaghan EG. Family pathways to child health. In: Amick BC III, Levine S, Tarlov AR, et al, editors. Society and health. New York: Oxford University Press; 1995. p. 18–45.
36. McClafferty H. Integrative pediatrics: looking forward. Children 2015;2(1):63–5.
37. Bethell CD, Hassink S, Abatemarco D, et al. Leveraging mind-body neuroscience and mindfulness to improve pediatrics. child and adolescent health measurement initiative mindfulness in pediatrics white paper initiative, 2012. Available at: http://beta.cahmi.org/wp-content/uploads/2013/12/Mindfulness-In-Pediatrics-and-MCH-Overview-Poster-Content-4_29_13-CB-1.pdf. Accessed October 10, 2015.
38. Gloria CT, Steinhardt MA. Relationships among positive emotions, coping, resilience and mental health. Stress Health 2014. [Epub ahead of print].

Child Maltreatment Prevention and the Scope of Child and Adolescent Psychiatry

John N. Constantino, MD

KEYWORDS

- Child • Maltreatment • Prevention • Psychiatry • Abuse • Neglect

KEY POINTS

- Child maltreatment is one of the most deleterious known influences on the mental health and development of children.
- A review of the risk variables associated with child maltreatment shows that the parents and caregivers of children at risk for maltreatment are commonly victims themselves. Their needs for social and psychiatric support are often easily ascertained in the early days of their children's lives, before catastrophic incidents of child maltreatment have occurred. Without these supports, child maltreatment continues to be the largest *preventable* causal influence on child mental disorder in the United States.
- It is incumbent on child and adolescent psychiatrists to know and ascertain the warning signs among the families of their patients, to recognize and exhaustively pursue opportunities for preventive intervention.
- For those children whose development is potentially compromised by the risk of child maltreatment, it is important that efforts to minimize such risk is sustained, comprehensive, and organized around the needs of individual families, not bureaucracies.
- In a next phase of development in our field, concerted efforts to learn which interventions work, when in the child's development, targeted toward whom, sustained at what dosage, and for what duration, will bring about cost-effective reductions in the incidence of child maltreatment and consequent improvement in major public mental health outcomes.

Funding Sources: This project was supported by grants from the Administration for Children and Families (90YR0054-04), the St. Louis County Children's Service Fund and an anonymous donor.
Conflict of Interest: Dr J.N. Constantino receives royalties from Western Psychological Services for commercial sales and distribution of the Social Responsiveness Scale-2, a quantitative measure of autistic traits that was not used in this report. The author otherwise has no competing financial interests.

Division of Child Psychiatry, Department of Psychiatry, Washington University School of Medicine, 660 South Euclid Avenue, Campus Box 8504, St Louis, MO 63110, USA
E-mail address: constantino@wustl.edu

Child Adolesc Psychiatric Clin N Am 25 (2016) 157–165
http://dx.doi.org/10.1016/j.chc.2015.11.003
1056-4993/16/$ – see front matter © 2016 The Author. Published by Elsevier Inc. This is an open access article under the CC BY-NC-ND license (http://creativecommons.org/licenses/by-nc-nd/4.0/).

Over the past 2 decades, a vast amount of knowledge has accrued regarding the prevalence and consequences of child maltreatment. The toll of these consequences has been confirmed in well-controlled, genetically informative studies showing that child maltreatment is one of the most deleterious known influences on the mental health and development of children.[1–4] Child maltreatment is preventable[5–7] but prevalent,[8] affecting at least 1 in 8 US children. The list of child and adolescent psychiatric conditions that are caused or exacerbated by child maltreatment is long, and it can be argued that of all of the influences on child mental disorders, most which are genetic,[9] child maltreatment is the single preventable cause with the highest associated disease burden, approaching 20% or more of the population-attributable risk for all psychiatric conditions of childhood.

Although there are important questions about the effectiveness of the steadily improving array of interventions designed to prevent child maltreatment, there is a need to engage a comprehensive approach to its prevention. There is no longer any question about whether child maltreatment contributes to the medical conditions of child psychiatry, and therefore a major share of the responsibility for the implementation of targeted (or secondary) child maltreatment prevention rests within the scope and science of child and adolescent psychiatry. For the same reasons that the prevention of lead poisoning advanced from the realm of public health departments (primary prevention) to its place in pediatric science and practice (targeted surveillance and prevention for patients at increased risk as identified by medical screening), it is no longer appropriate for child maltreatment prevention to be relegated exclusively to state departments of social services. Furthermore, the threshold for physician engagement must move beyond imminent risk (ie, calls to state child abuse/neglect hotline) to more sophisticated appraisals of highly prevalent risk scenarios that are between the respective scopes of universal primary prevention efforts and emergency intervention by municipal courts after an incidence of abuse or neglect has already occurred. As a clinical determinant of disease, one for which the predictors and consequences are uniquely encountered in child psychiatric practice, child maltreatment in the United States (and many other high-income countries) belongs to child and adolescent psychiatry.

This article briefly reviews a complement of methods that are ready to incorporate into child and adolescent psychiatric practice, by virtue of having established a reasonable evidence base (to be considered an imperfect but necessary starting point). The interventions proposed here have been validated either with respect to the prevention of child maltreatment or with respect to adverse outcomes associated with maltreatment (and primarily focused on enhancing the caregiving environment); they are feasible for integration into clinical decision making, and, most importantly, can be included in the training of the next generation of clinicians. They are summarized in **Box 1**. However, in relation to the prospect of expanding practice, few if any of these interventions are (or need to be) routinely performed by child psychiatrists alone, but, as with referral to a specialist for electroconvulsive therapy (ECT) or cognitive-behavioral therapy, they involve collaborations through which long-term risk for child maltreatment can be managed. This article does not assert that this set of interventions is new or should be restricted to the practice of child psychiatry (there are many disciplines to credit for their development), or that these interventions have never been included in child psychiatric practice. Instead it responds to the state of science, recognizing that not enough is currently done to prepare or equip child and adolescent psychiatrists to implement or advocate for this set of clinical interventions for the families of their patients. In many practice settings, some or all of these

---

Box 1
Elements of evidence-based practice relevant to the prevention of child maltreatment

Ascertainment of robust predictors of child maltreatment

Home visitation for infant/toddler siblings of selected child psychiatric patients

Evidence-based parenting education

Surrogate caregiving (including high-quality early childhood education and multidimensional treatment foster care)

Parent-child interactional therapy (preventive)

Bullying prevention

In-home case management (preventive)

Two-generation psychiatric care

---

methods are unavailable, inaccessible, or unreimbursed. This unacceptable reality is unlikely to change if the interventions are not accessed whenever possible, used to advantage, and advocated by physicians.

APPRAISAL OF RISK FOR CHILD MALTREATMENT

Large-scale studies of family and environmental factors that index risk for officially reported child maltreatment have clarified that a short list of variables represent compelling indications for enhanced surveillance and targeted approaches to maltreatment prevention. The extent to which the presence of these factors raises risk is amplified when they co-occur and by the condition of poverty, which affects some 32% of all US children, and with which many of these factors are correlated. Leading predictors are summarized with citations in **Box 2**. Inventories of these factors have been devised and tested for the ability to specify actionable levels of risk for child maltreatment.[10] As an example of the predictive power of combining 2 risk factors, among Missouri

---

Box 2
Readily identifiable indicators of increased risk for child maltreatment

Prior history of maltreatment of a child[11]

Poverty[12]

Parental history of placement in foster care[13]

Unintended pregnancy[14]

Intimate partner violence[15]

Parental mental health condition[16,17]
- Psychiatric disorders[18]
- Substance use disorders
- Developmental disorders

Neighborhood characteristics related to access to early childhood education, mental health, and social services[19–21]

Family size[22]

Temperamental characteristics of infants (so-called fussy babies"; see Barr,[23] 2014)

Data from Refs.[11–23]

---

offspring of parents with alcohol use disorders enrolled in the Collaborative Study on the Genetics of Alcoholism (COGA), Jonson-Reid and colleagues[4] reported that the proportion identified in the state official-report registry for child abuse was 57% for those whose family incomes were below the federal poverty line versus 7% for their counterparts above the federal poverty line. Accumulations of more than 2 risk factors, many of which can be reliably ascertained on the first day of an infant's life, have resulted in predictions of even higher proportions of children ultimately maltreated.

Home Visitation for Infant/Toddler Patients and Infant/Toddler Siblings of Patients

For families identified by child psychiatrists with any of the risk factors discussed earlier, and in which there resides an infant (aged birth to 3 years), a case can be made that a referral for nurse home visitation is indicated.[24–27] There are numerous models for the delivery of home visitation; they vary with respect to profession of the home visitor (nurse vs case manager vs other paraprofessional), specific populations to which they are tailored, and demonstrated effectiveness for reducing child maltreatment. For a recent exhaustive analysis, entitled *Home Visiting Evidence of Effectiveness Review*, see US Office of Planning, Research and Evaluation Report #2014-59 (http://homvee.acf.hhs.gov/HomVEE_Executive_Summary_2014-59.pdf). The Nurse Family Partnership model advanced by David Olds and colleagues (2014)[5] has achieved the strongest evidence base with 1 order of magnitude reductions in the incidence of child maltreatment among at-risk groups, but the studies to date have largely been restricted to families with firstborn infants (see also Lanier and Jonson-Reid,[28] 2014). Despite (1) the growing availability of nurse home visitation programs nationally, (2) the current prevalence of child maltreatment, (3) the high frequency with which risk factors for child maltreatment are encountered by clinicians, (4) the availability of methods for the engagement of families at risk in preventive interventions such as home visitation,[29] and (5) the increasingly documented impact of the intervention, the proportion of all US children in the 2011 to 2012 birth cohort who did not receive a single home visit during the first 3 years of life was 86% (http://datacenter.kidscount.org/). These statistics delineate lost opportunity for child maltreatment prevention. At present it is rare for successful referrals to home visitation to be initiated by mental health specialists (as opposed to providers of primary obstetric, newborn medicine, and pediatric care) despite child psychiatric populations being highly enriched (more so than any other medical specialty) for young families at combined inherited and environmental risk for child maltreatment and its consequences.

Evidence-Based Parenting Education and Parent-Child Interactional Therapy

Although the current generation of evidence-based parent training programs have yet to be systematically assessed with respect to the prevention of child maltreatment per se, it stands to reason that those that effectively prevent or reduce clinical behavioral abnormalities in children (see Presnall and colleagues,[30] 2014) should necessarily reduce maltreatment risk because they are centered on the modification of maladaptive parenting behavior. Among evidence-based parenting education programs, the 2 that have shown the most promise for child maltreatment prevention are Triple P, an intervention that is scaled to the needs and risk level of each individual family (see Prinz and colleagues[31] for a promising large-scale study, conducted by the developers of the intervention, of impact on maltreatment) and The Incredible Years, a group-based parenting education program (see Hurlburt and colleagues[32] for description of a trial among families that self-reported child maltreatment). These and other evidence-based parent training curricula are becoming increasingly available nationwide, but are rarely systematically implemented in child psychiatric practice. An extensively validated therapeutic variation on the theme of parent training, parent-child interactional therapy, has steadily gained traction as a standard facet of treatment of young children manifesting clinical behavioral abnormalities; a recent innovative analysis of the utility of the intervention for child maltreatment prevention was very promising and warrants replication.[22]

Other Evidence-Based Interventions in the Prevention of Child Maltreatment

When primary caregivers have limitations in their ability to ensure around-the-clock safety to children under their care, surrogate caregiving environments, including high-quality child care and foster care, become lifelines for families. These expensive propositions are often reserved for the aftermath of a first incidence of abuse or neglect, but novel interventions that enhance the level of sensitive-responsive care by surrogates in such environments are proving capable of promoting resilience in youth at risk and improved outcomes for their families.[33] Note that, in a large administrative-data study of chronic, official-report child abuse or neglect, Jonson-Reid and colleagues[34] showed that children who experienced a single episode of official-report maltreatment, but no further occurrences, incurred rates of mental health care use that were not significantly increased compared with those of children in the general population. Thus, interventions designed to prevent child maltreatment recidivism (discussed later) are as important and potentially potent as those that are designed to prevent its initial incidence. Kessler and colleagues[35] showed significant reductions in adult mental disorders among foster care alumni (primarily school aged) who had been assigned to a model program in which their case managers had higher levels of training and lower caseloads than was customary for usual foster care. The outcomes of other efforts to enhance the foster caregiving environment (eg, via multi-dimensional treatment foster care, a wrap-around multimodal intervention for foster families of children and adolescents with challenging behavior) have been promising and warrant further study.[35,36]

In general, the proactive implementation of case management services for families at risk (ie, before maltreatment occurs rather than afterward) has garnered a growing evidence base[37–40] and should become a high priority for conversion from its currently exclusive role in treatment to a role in targeted preventive intervention. The reduction of risk for maltreatment outside of primary caregiving environments is best exemplified by manualized bullying prevention curricula, which, despite free access (http://www.stopbullying.gov/) and a large evidence base documenting unequivocal impact, remain underutilized and not familiar enough to practicing child and adolescent psychiatrists.

In addition, more than a decade ago, Zeanah and colleagues[41] reported on the naturalistic results of a family court collaboration with an academic division of child psychiatry (Tulane University, New Orleans, LA), in which child psychiatrists with expertise in infancy participated in the disposition planning and support of young children in foster care. The program, which has been continuously subsidized by local government funding to the present time, conducts serial, comprehensive appraisals of health, mental health, and social factors that influence risk for abuse and neglect recidivism in each case. Notably, the clinicians deliver regularly updated intervention recommendations to the court, and these include specifications regarding safety of visitation, the provision of mental health treatment to birth parents whenever necessary, continuous appraisal of the quality of the parent-child relationship, and ultimately comprehensive medical recommendations to the court detailing necessary parameters and supports for safe reunification. The program reduced (by more than half) the occurrence of maltreatment recidivism compared with a matched group of children who did not receive the intervention. A recent attempt to replicate the Tulane approach for young children at extreme high risk resulted in similarly low levels of child maltreatment recidivism.[16] The program serves as a prototype for what are currently referred to as two-generation interventions; other successful examples are described by Shonkoff and Fisher,[42] and the effectiveness of treatment of parental mental health conditions on the outcomes of children was recently reviewed in an important meta-analysis conducted by Siegenthaler and colleagues.[43]

SUMMARY AND FUTURE DIRECTIONS

A review of the risk variables associated with child maltreatment highlight that the parents and caregivers of children at risk for maltreatment are themselves victims. They are in need of programs that are increasingly available and well established. Their needs for those supports are often easily ascertained in the early days of their children's lives, before catastrophic incidents of child maltreatment have occurred. Without these supports child maltreatment continues to be the largest preventable causal influence on child mental disorder in the United States. It is thus incumbent on child and adolescent psychiatrists to know and ascertain the warning signs among the families of their patients, to recognize and exhaustively pursue opportunities for preventive intervention. To do this they should become experts in the emerging science of child maltreatment prevention.

Note that in child psychiatry there is rarely such a thing as a one-time inoculation against mental disorder, or, for that matter, against maltreatment. Behavior is complex, adaptive, and highly evolved (with many checks and balances). Often when things go awry the causes are multifactorial. For those children whose development is potentially compromised by the risk of child maltreatment, it is important that efforts to minimize such risk are sustained, comprehensive, and organized around the needs of individual families, not bureaucracies.

The current generation of specialists in child mental health, clinicians and researchers alike, need to be trained in these methods and to be integral proponents of the advancing frontier of preventive intervention.[44] In the next phase of development, concerted efforts to learn which interventions work, when in the child's development, targeted toward whom, sustained at what dosage, and for what duration, will bring about cost-effective reductions in the incidence of child maltreatment and consequent improvement in major public mental health outcomes. Embedding such intervention efforts in genetically and/or developmentally informative sampling designs with robust outcome measurements will ensure that the agenda of separating "baby from bathwater" in preventive intervention will itself contribute to the steady advancement of behavioral neuroscience.

REFERENCES

1. Binder EB, Bradley RG, Liu W, et al. Association of FKBP5 polymorphisms and childhood abuse with risk of posttraumatic stress disorder symptoms in adults. JAMA 2008;299(11):1291–305.
2. Gilbert R, Widom CS, Browne K, et al. Burden and consequences of child maltreatment in high-income countries. Lancet 2009;373(9657):68–81.
3. Horan JM, Widom CS. From childhood maltreatment to allostatic load in adulthood: the role of social support. Child Maltreat 2015;20(4):229–39.
4. Jonson-Reid M, Presnall N, Drake B, et al. The effects of child maltreatment and inherited liability on antisocial development: an official records study. J Am Acad Child Adolesc Psychiatry 2010;49(4):321–32.

5. Donelan-McCall N, Eckenrode J, Olds DL. Home visiting for the prevention of child maltreatment: lessons learned during the past 20 years. Pediatr Clin North Am 2009;56(2):389–403.
6. Knerr W, Gardner F, Cluver L. Improving positive parenting skills and reducing harsh and abusive parenting in low- and middle-income countries: a systematic review. Prev Sci 2013;14(4):352–63.
7. Selph SS, Bougatsos C, Blazina I, et al. Behavioral interventions and counseling to prevent child abuse and neglect: a systematic review to update the US preventive services task force recommendation. Ann Intern Med 2013;158(3):179–90.
8. Wildeman C, Emanuel N, Leventhal JM, et al. The prevalence of confirmed maltreatment among US children, 2004 to 2011. JAMA Pediatr 2014;168(8):706–13.
9. Kendler KS. What psychiatric genetics has taught us about the nature of psychiatric illness and what is left to learn. Mol Psychiatry 2013;18(10):1058–66.
10. Diderich HM, Fekkes M, Verkerk PH, et al. A new protocol for screening adults presenting with their own medical problems at the emergency department to identify children at high risk for maltreatment. Child Abuse Negl 2013;37(12):1122–31.
11. Jonson-Reid M. Foster care and future risk of maltreatment. Child Youth Serv Rev 2003;25(4):271–94.
12. Jonson-Reid M, Drake B, Zhou P. Neglect subtypes, race, and poverty: individual, family, and service characteristics. Child Maltreat 2013;18(1):30–41.
13. Dworsky A. Child welfare services involvement among the children of young parents in foster care. Child Abuse Negl 2015;45:68–79.
14. Guterman K. Unintended pregnancy as a predictor of child maltreatment. Child Abuse Negl 2015;48:160–9.
15. Connelly CD, Hazen AL, Coben JH, et al. Persistence of intimate partner violence among families referred to child welfare. J Interpers Violence 2006;21(6):774–97.
16. Constantino JN. Two-generation psychiatric intervention in the prevention of early childhood maltreatment recidivism. Am J Psychiatry 2016, in press.
17. O'Donnell M, Maclean MJ, Sims S, et al. Maternal mental health and risk of child protection involvement: mental health diagnoses associated with increased risk. J Epidemiol Community Health 2015;69(12):1175–83.
18. Chuang E, Wells R, Aarons GA. Identifying depression in a national sample of caregivers investigated in regard to their child's welfare. Psychiatr Serv 2014;65(7):911–7.
19. Afifi TO, Taillieu T, Cheung K, et al. Substantiated reports of child maltreatment from the Canadian Incidence Study of Reported Child Abuse and Neglect 2008: examining child and household characteristics and child functional impairment. Can J Psychiatry 2015;60(7):315–23.
20. Klein S. The availability of neighborhood early care and education resources and the maltreatment of young children. Child Maltreat 2011;16(4):300–11.
21. Maguire-Jack K, Klein S. Parenting and proximity to social services: lessons from Los Angeles County in the community context of child neglect. Child Abuse Negl 2015;45:35–45.
22. Lanier P, Kohl PL, Benz J, et al. Preventing maltreatment with a community-based implementation of parent-child interaction therapy. J Child Fam Stud 2014;23(2):449–60.
23. Barr RG. Crying as a trigger for abusive head trauma: a key to prevention. Pediatr Radiol 2014;44(Suppl 4):S559–s564.

24. Chaffin M, Hecht D, Bard D, et al. A statewide trial of the SafeCare home-based services model with parents in child protective services. Pediatrics 2012;129(3): 509–15.

25. Cowart-Osborne M, Jackson M, Chege E, et al. Technology-based innovations in child maltreatment prevention programs: examples from SafeCare®. Soc Sci (Basel) 2014;3(3):427–40.

26. Miller TR. Projected outcomes of nurse-family partnership home visitation during 1996-2013, USA. Prev Sci 2015;16(6):765–77.

27. Sumner SA, Mercy JA, Dahlberg LL, et al. Violence in the United States: status, challenges, and opportunities. JAMA 2015;314(5):478–88.

28. Lanier P, Jonson-Reid M. Comparing primiparous and multiparous mothers in a nurse home visiting prevention program. Birth 2014;41(4):344–52.

29. Constantino JN. Child mental health: status of the promise, the reality, and the future of prevention. In: Cottler LB, editor. Mental health in public health: the next 100 years. Oxford (United Kingdom): Oxford University Press; 2011. p. xvii, 348.

30. Presnall N, Webster-Stratton CH, Constantino JN. Parent training: equivalent improvement in externalizing behavior for children with and without familial risk. J Am Acad Child Adolesc Psychiatry 2014;53(8):879–87, 887.e1–2.

31. Prinz RJ, Sanders MR, Shapiro CJ, et al. Population based prevention of child maltreatment: the US Triple P system population trial. Prev Sci 2009;10:1–12.

32. Hurlburt MS, Nguyen K, Reid J, et al. Efficacy of the Incredible Years group parent program with families in Head Start who self-reported a history of child maltreatment. Child Abuse Negl 2013;37(8):531–43.

33. Leve LD, Harold GT, Chamberlain P, et al. Practitioner review: children in foster care–vulnerabilities and evidence-based interventions that promote resilience processes. J Child Psychol Psychiatry 2012;53(12):1197–211.

34. Jonson-Reid M, Kohl PL, Drake B. Child and adult outcomes of chronic child maltreatment. Pediatrics 2012;129(5):839–45.

35. Kessler RC, Pecora PJ, Williams J, et al. Effects of enhanced foster care on the long-term physical and mental health of foster care alumni. Arch Gen Psychiatry 2008;65(6):625–33.

36. Leve LD, Kerr DC, Harold GT. Young adult outcomes associated with teen pregnancy among high-risk girls in an RCT of multidimensional treatment foster care. J Child Adolesc Subst Abuse 2013;22(5):421–34.

37. Dubowitz H, Feigelman S, Lane W, et al. Pediatric primary care to help prevent child maltreatment: the Safe Environment for Every Kid (SEEK) model. Pediatrics 2009;123(3):858–64.

38. Guterman NB, Tabone JK, Bryan GM, et al. Examining the effectiveness of home-based parent aide services to reduce risk for physical child abuse and neglect: six-month findings from a randomized clinical trial. Child Abuse Negl 2013;37(8): 566–77.

39. May PA, Marais AS, Gossage JP, et al. Case management reduces drinking during pregnancy among high risk women. Int J Alcohol Drug Res 2013;2(3):61–70.

40. Slesnick N, Erdem G. Efficacy of ecologically-based treatment with substance-abusing homeless mothers: substance use and housing outcomes. J Subst Abuse Treat 2013;45(5):416–25.

41. Zeanah CH, Larrieu JA, Heller SS, et al. Evaluation of a preventive intervention for maltreated infants and toddlers in foster care. J Am Acad Child Adolesc Psychiatry 2001;40(2):214–21.

42. Shonkoff JP, Fisher PA. Rethinking evidence-based practice and two-generation programs to create the future of early childhood policy. Dev Psychopathol 2013; 25(4 Pt 2):1635–53.

43. Siegenthaler E, Munder T, Egger M. Effect of preventive interventions in mentally ill parents on the mental health of the offspring: systematic review and meta-analysis. J Am Acad Child Adolesc Psychiatry 2012;51(1):8–17.e8.

44. Shoemaker EZ, Tully LM, Niendam TA, et al. The next big thing in child and adolescent psychiatry: interventions to prevent and intervene early in psychiatric illnesses. Psychiatr Clin North Am 2015;38(3):475–94.

The Vermont Family Based Approach

Family Based Health Promotion, Illness Prevention, and Intervention

Jim Hudziak, MD*, Masha Y. Ivanova, PhD

KEYWORDS

- Vermont family based approach • VFBA • Family Wellness Coaching
- Focused Family Coaching • Innovative healthcare
- Family based emotional and behavioral healthcare

KEY POINTS

- Because all health is tied to emotional and behavioral health, we need innovative healthcare approaches that target emotional and behavioral health to improve general health.
- The Vermont Family Based Approach (VFBA) is a healthcare paradigm that aims to improve population health by improving emotional and behavioral health.
- Because the family is a powerful health-promoting social institution, the VFBA also aims to shift the delivery of healthcare to the family level.
- Based on the results of a comprehensive family based assessment of health and family functioning, the VFBA offers evidence-based health promotion, prevention, and intervention to the entire family.
- All families are partnered with Family Wellness Coaches to implement a comprehensive program of health and wellness. Where indicated, families are also partnered with focused family coaches (family based psychotherapists) and family based psychiatrists.

INTRODUCTION

All health is tied to emotional and behavioral health. Emotional and behavioral problems directly predict or influence the course of major nonpsychiatric medical conditions.[1] In contrast, positive affective states are associated with physical health.[2,3] To improve population health, we need innovative approaches to healthcare that target emotional and behavioral health.

This article introduces the Vermont Family Based Approach (VFBA[4]), a healthcare paradigm that aims to improve population health by improving emotional and

Department of Psychiatry, University of Vermont College of Medicine & University of Vermont Medical Center, 1 South Prospect Street, Burlington, VT 05495, USA
* Corresponding author.
E-mail address: James.Hudziak@uvm.edu

Child Adolesc Psychiatric Clin N Am 25 (2016) 167–178
http://dx.doi.org/10.1016/j.chc.2015.11.002   **childpsych.theclinics.com**
1056-4993/16/$ – see front matter © 2016 Elsevier Inc. All rights reserved.

behavioral health. Equally important, the VFBA aims to shift the delivery of health-care to the family level. This is because health is familial in nature, or "runs" in families. Families have health-related attitudes, beliefs, and practices that are shared among family members and passed through generations.[5,6] The family is the primary health system, an influential social institution with health-promoting power.

This article also offers the empirical argument for the VFBA, which is set in the context of the early childhood period (defined as birth to age 5), one of the many critical periods for health promotion and prevention.

THE VERMONT FAMILY BASED APPROACH

The VFBA uses evidence-based health promotion, prevention, and intervention from the family perspective (**Fig. 1**). It emphasizes the importance of emotional and behavioral health for health in general, recognizes parental emotional and behavioral health as essential for children's health, and individualizes evidence-based care to meet the unique needs of each family. The VFBA also emphasizes the early childhood period as a critical intervention point because preventing problems from developing in the first place or treating them before they become intractable can avert suffering, improve healthcare outcomes, and reduce healthcare costs.

As the strongest predictors of morbidity and mortality among all health conditions, emotional and behavioral problems are a serious societal burden. Except for their most severe manifestations, emotional and behavioral problems are also invisible to the naked eye. Because they are socially costly and often invisible, they should be regularly assessed using psychometrically sound, standardized assessment instruments. Routine, population-wide screening of emotional and behavioral health could also help to de-stigmatize emotional and behavioral difficulties.

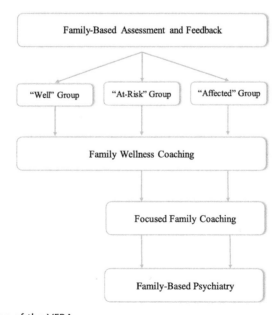

Fig. 1. Illustration of the VFBA.

The VFBA starts with a comprehensive, family based assessment of emotional and behavioral health. Both children and parents receive direct, empirically based assessment of their emotional and behavioral strengths and difficulties. The typical VFBA family assessment includes assessment of each family member's emotional and behavioral health, family routines and practices, parenting, enrichment activities, and family relationships. Families are offered results of their family based assessment using the Family Assessment and Feedback Intervention (FAFI),[7] a brief, family based therapeutic assessment feedback intervention.

Based on the results of the VFBA family based assessment, families are classified into the "Well," "At-Risk," and "Affected" groups. "Well" families are defined as families in which neither parents nor children experience significant emotional and behavioral problems, "At-Risk" families are families in which parents but not children experience significant emotional and behavioral problems, thus putting their children's development at risk through both genetic and environmental influence. Families are assigned to the "Affected" group if the children (and possibly parents) are experiencing significant emotional and behavioral problems.

Following this assessment-based classification, families are engaged in the VFBA at different programmatic levels: all families receive support in achieving and maintaining wellness. In addition, families assigned to the "At-Risk" and "Affected" groups receive more specialized, therapeutic services.

Vermont Family Based Approach Family Wellness Coaching

Most parents do not receive any formal training in raising healthy and happy children, and model their parenting after the care they received from their own parents. Meanwhile, there is strong empirical evidence that specific parenting behaviors predict positive child development. These include health-promoting family routines and practices (eg, mealtime and bedtime routines, limited screen time) and positive discipline techniques (eg, rewarding appropriate behavior, ignoring mild misbehavior). To offer parents training and ongoing support in raising healthy children, families are partnered with family wellness coaches (FWCs). An FWC is a bachelor's- or master's-level health or education professional who is trained in a range of evidence-based approaches to motivational enhancement, family based assessment, health-promoting family routines and practices, and positive parenting, as well as exercise, nutrition, and music engagement. Each family, regardless of its group assignment, is partnered with a FWC, which is the universal or primary prevention element of the model.

Guided by the unique results of each family's VFBA assessment, the FWC helps the family to devise and implement a comprehensive, individualized program of health and wellness. To strengthen family engagement in the VFBA program, the FWCs often start their partnerships with families by arranging health-promotion activities for the children (eg, music lessons, exercise classes) at no or reduced cost to the family. The FWC then helps the parents to set up health-promoting family routines so that family members get sufficient sleep, exercise, and healthy food. As part of this work, the FWC may teach parents how to shop for healthy ingredients, cook nutritious meals, and minimize electronic screen exposure. The FWC also may help parents to develop positive discipline strategies and emotion regulation skills (eg, mindfulness, relaxation, purposeful distraction). Furthermore, the FWC may assist families in solving the challenges of daily living, such as housing, food access, or transportation problems.

If results of family based assessment indicate that the parents ("At-Risk" group) or children ("Affected" group) suffer from significant emotional and behavioral problems, the family is also partnered with an focused family coach, as described below.

Vermont Family Based Approach Focused Family Coaching

Emotional and behavioral health professionals working with children commonly acknowledge that their efforts to help children would be more effective if they could also improve the emotional and behavioral health of the children's parents. Because parents create the environments in which the children develop and parental emotional and behavioral problems disrupt parenting, the VFBA stresses the importance of treating parental emotional and behavioral problems to ensure healthy child outcomes. The family focus of the VFBA provides a natural context for the conversation about the parents' own emotional and behavioral difficulties. Our clinical experiences suggest that openly discussing with the parents that their emotional and behavioral health is crucial for their children's successful development enhances the parents' engagement in their own emotional and behavioral treatment.

A focused family coach (FFC) is a licensed master's- or doctoral-level psychotherapist who provides evidence-based psychotherapeutic interventions from the family perspective. An FFC operates from the family perspective in 2 ways: first, a FFC assesses the emotional and behavioral health of all family members and, where appropriate, devises a psychotherapeutic treatment for all family members. Second, when devising a psychotherapeutic intervention, a FFC selects family based evidence-based interventions where those are available, or adapts existing evidence-based interventions developed for individual treatment to be applied from the family perspective.

Where indicated, families are also partnered with a family based psychiatrist, in part to determine the appropriateness of a psychopharmacological intervention to augment family based health promotion and psychotherapy. Partnering "At-Risk" families (where parents but not children experience emotional and behavioral problems) with FFCs and family based psychiatrists constitutes the secondary prevention aspect of the VFBA.

Vermont Family Based Approach Psychiatry

Over the past half a century, psychiatry has become confined to the understanding and treatment of severe psychiatric disorders. In the VFBA, the family based psychiatrist works with other members of the VFBA team to interpret the results of the family based assessment, design and implement the family's comprehensive program of health and wellness. The psychiatrist's scope of practice is thus expanded beyond severe psychiatric disorders to the full spectrum of emotional and behavioral functioning. Moreover, the VFBA family based psychiatrists are trained in evidence-based health promotion, prevention, and psychotherapeutic interventions in addition to their training in pharmacotherapy.

In the same way that cardiologists do not circumscribe their professional scope to end-stage cardiovascular disease, but design heart-healthy health promotion and prevention approaches for population-wide cardiovascular health, the VFBA psychiatrists do not circumscribe their professional scope to severe psychiatric conditions, but design brain-healthy health promotion and prevention approaches for population-wide emotional and behavioral health.

The Vermont Family Based Approach in Community Settings

A pilot VFBA project demonstrated its feasibility and acceptability in an urban Head Start program in Sioux Falls, South Dakota (Stanger S, Ivanova MY, Hall A, et al. School-based family wellness: A gateway to service utilization. Submitted for publication). A randomized trial of the VFBA is currently under way in a pediatric clinic. It aims to establish the feasibility and acceptability of the VFBA and test its efficacy with families of young children. Families of 3- to 6-year-olds are being randomized to receive either the VFBA or pediatric care as usual. Families in the VFBA group are receiving the comprehensive VFBA assessment, therapeutic assessment feedback via the FAFI,[7] a partnership with an FWC, as well as support from an FFC and family based psychiatrists, if needed. Children in the VFBA group are also receiving music training, while their parents receive a group behavioral parent training intervention during the children's music lessons.

In the following, we review several key empirical findings that informed the VFBA, focusing on the early childhood period. Consistent with this issue's emphasis on population health, our review emphasizes studies conducted with families in the general population.

THE CASE FOR THE VERMONT FAMILY BASED APPROACH
Family Routines and Practices are Mechanisms of Health Promotion

Every day parents of young children engage in family routines and practices that have powerful health consequences, such as morning, bedtime, and evening routines; grocery shopping; and food preparation. Although these routines and practices comprise the fundamental matrix of family life, few parents receive any training in providing them.

Interventions that enhance health-promoting family routines and practices have been found effective with families of young children. For example, Mindell and colleagues[8] reviewed 52 intervention trials for children's sleep problems that were conducted with parents of young children. All trials occurred in the general population and tested behavioral interventions targeting parenting practices (eg, how to create a soothing bedtime routine, ignore noncompliant behavior, stay consistent). Behavioral parenting interventions produced significant reductions in children's bedtime resistance and night wakings in 49 (94%) of the 52 trials.

As part of a broader review of intervention studies for reducing screen time, Schmidt and colleagues[9] reported the results of 9 trials that targeted parenting practices in families with young children. Interventions were delivered in family homes or primary care clinics mostly in families preselected for low socioeconomic status or high child body mass index (BMI). Eight (89%) of the 9 studies reported significant positive effects on such health-related outcomes as child and parent TV viewing, child video-game playing, child BMI, parental self-efficacy, and behavioral efforts for minimizing children's screen exposure. All 8 studies that supported the effectiveness of the interventions involved a health professional or paraprofessional directly working with the parents to change their family routines and practices. The only study that did not show a significant effect lacked this relational component, as it used mailings of educational newsletters to families.

Parents of young children can be coached to provide health-promoting family routines and practices. The reviewed interventions changed parenting behavior, which in turn changed health-related child outcomes, such as sleep quality and BMI. The review by Schmidt and colleagues[9] also suggested that parenting practices are more likely to change when the intervention includes face-to-face parent coaching by a member of the intervention team.

In the VFBA, the FWC establishes a close relationship with families and works with them to develop health-promoting family routines and practices. The FWCs are essential for catalyzing, sustaining, and generalizing behavior change for families.

Positive Parenting Promotes Children's Health

Although it is certainly exciting, the early childhood period also can be challenging for parents as a time of grueling schedules and rapid transitions. Ineffective parenting styles get established during this period and gain traction as the child and family develop. Fortunately, there is overwhelming empirical evidence that behavioral parent training interventions can help parents of young children to build long-lasting positive parenting skills.

The most well-researched behavioral parent training programs for parents of young children are *Helping the Noncompliant Child*,[10] *Incredible Years*,[11] *Parent Management Training*,[12] and *Triple-P*.[13] Based on social learning principles, these approaches teach parents specific behaviors that increase their children's compliance and prosocial behavior and reduce oppositional and aggressive behavior.

Behavioral parent training programs were developed as clinical interventions for children with externalizing behavior problems, such as oppositional, disruptive, and aggressive behavior. As part of a meta-analytic review of 79 clinical trials with families of children and adolescents, Maughan and colleagues[14] reported the efficacy of behavioral parent training interventions specifically for 3-year-olds to 5-year-olds (number of studies not reported). The effect size of the intervention on children's behavior problems was medium for studies with between-subjects designs (Cohen $d = 0.40$) and large for studies with within-subject designs (Cohen $d = 0.75$). As part of another meta-analytic review that included only between-subjects designs, Lundahl and colleagues[15] also estimated the effect size for behavior problems to be medium (Cohen $d = 0.44$). It was somewhat larger for observed (Cohen $d = 0.48$) and self-reported (Cohen $d = 0.45$) parenting competency.

There is thus strong evidence that behavioral parent training interventions are effective in clinical trials with families of children who already display externalizing problems. Dishion and colleagues[16] tested whether behavioral training interventions could also be applied in population-wide prevention trials using their Family Check-Up intervention.

The Family Check-Up is a 3-session assessment and feedback intervention that involves assessment of parent-child interactions from the perspective of behavioral parent training, and giving parents feedback about the results of their assessment using motivational enhancement strategies.[17] The goal of the Family Check-Up is to identify problematic parenting practices and enhance the parents' willingness to engage in behavioral parent training to learn more positive parenting techniques to ultimately reduce children's externalizing problems. A total of 731 families who were enrolled in the Women, Infants, and Children (WIC) nutritional supplement program were randomly assigned to receive the Family Check-Up when the children were 2, 3, and 4 years old or to continue their participation in the WIC program as usual. The Family Check-Up intervention was associated with a slower increase of children's externalizing problem behavior over the 2-year span of the study. This effect was maintained over the subsequent 3-year follow-up period, when the children were assessed in elementary school.[18]

Behavioral parent training interventions are effective for reducing the externalizing behavior problems of young children. A large body of evidence indicates that they can be applied with young children who are already displaying significant externalizing behavior problems. Results obtained by Dishion and colleagues[16] also indicate that behavioral parent training interventions can be applied with families of young children in the general population, where children may or may not be displaying externalizing problems. From the perspective of population health, work by Dishion and colleagues[16] indicates that a short version of a behavioral parent training intervention in the framework of therapeutic assessment feedback can produce long-lasting results.

The VFBA includes family based therapeutic assessment feedback, which is delivered via the FAFI[7] discussed earlier. The FAFI presents the results of the broad VFBA family assessment, including assessment of parenting practices. As part of the VFBA, FWCs also work with all families from the perspective of behavioral parent training to help parents develop positive parenting skills. When the results of family based assessment indicate that a more intensive behavioral parent training intervention is needed, FFCs provide it to families.

Parental Emotional/Behavioral Health Is Essential for Children's Healthy Development

Parental emotional/behavioral health is essential for a healthy family environment. Berg-Nielsen and colleagues[19] reviewed studies testing the association between parental emotional and behavioral health and parenting across childhood, concluding that parental emotional and behavioral health difficulties significantly impair the quality of parenting. The investigators also concluded that the primary parenting challenges faced by parents with significant emotional and behavioral difficulties are heightened negativity toward the child and ineffective discipline practices.

Several studies have examined the association between parental emotional and behavioral health and children's developmental outcomes in families with young children. Zajicek-Farber and colleagues[20] tested relations among maternal depressive symptoms, parenting stress, engagement in bedtime routines and children's emotional and behavioral regulation among 2977 families enrolled in the Early Head Start Research and Evaluation project. Maternal self-reported depressive symptoms negatively affected children's investigator-rated emotional and behavioral regulation via 2 pathways. In the first pathway, maternal depression exacerbated maternal stress, which weakened children's emotional and behavioral regulation. In the second pathway, maternal stress also weakened maternal engagement with bedtime routines, which weakened children's emotional and behavioral regulation.

Hur and colleagues[21] reported similar findings in their study of 444 families with preschoolers who were recruited from early child-care and education programs. Most parents were mothers (89%), and all data were based on parental reports. The study tested relations among parental depressive symptoms, children's socioemotional development, and family chaos, defined as the degree of disorganization in the home. Family chaos mediated the influence of parental depressive symptoms on children's socioemotional development, while controlling for child age, gender, race/ethnicity, number of children in the home, parental marital status, and family income.

Parental emotional and behavioral health is important for the creation of a health-promoting family environment. When parents struggle with emotional/behavioral problems, it challenges their ability to discipline their children effectively,[19] and to provide health-promoting family routines and practices.[20,21] This suggests that healthcare efforts supporting young children should directly focus on parental emotional and behavioral health.

Direct assessment and support of parental emotional/behavioral health is a cornerstone of the VFBA. All members of a VFBA team, including FWCs, FFCs, and family based psychiatrists, are trained to apply evidence-based health promotion, prevention, and intervention strategies to address the emotional and behavioral health of both children and their parents.

Enrichment Activities Promote Children's Health

Well families are families where parents and children not only sit down for family dinner and go to bed on time, but also enjoy individual and family enrichment activities. The literature on the health benefits of enrichment activities for young children is only beginning to emerge, and our review focuses on the 2 activities that have received the most attention.

Contemplative interventions

Greenberg and Harris[22] reviewed empirical studies testing the health-promoting effects of contemplative practices for children and adolescents. Contemplative practices were defined as "structured activities requiring volitional control over physical and mental activity" (p. 162). Most of the reviewed studies focused on contemplative practices for older children and adolescents. Greenberg and Harris concluded that contemplative interventions have shown some benefits in both universal prevention and clinical trials. Across studies, contemplative interventions were associated with children's enhanced self-regulation and improved social and academic functioning. The authors also cautioned, however, that the high enthusiasm for contemplative interventions overshadowed the empirical evidence available for them.

Two recent prevention trials with preschoolers have supported the findings by Greenberg and Harris[22] for young children. Fisak[23] reported results of a small parent-focused trial of an anxiety-prevention program for shy preschoolers. Eighteen parents received a 10-session group intervention that comprised a traditional behavioral parent-training curriculum, plus a mindful parenting intervention. The mindful parenting intervention coached parents in the nonjudgmental awareness of moment-by-moment experiences, acceptance of internal events, and psychological distancing. The program was acceptable to the parents and associated with a reduction in children's parent-reported shyness and behavioral inhibition. Although the results of this trial are promising, its design makes it impossible to determine the unique effects of the mindfulness intervention.

Flook and colleagues[24] conducted a school-based randomized trial of a mindfulness-based Kindness Curriculum with 68 preschoolers. The 12-week Kindness Curriculum comprised "children's literature, music, and movement to teach and stabilize concepts related to kindness and compassion." (p. 45). It was delivered to the entire classroom as part of a regular school day twice a week for 20 to 30 minutes. Over the course of the trial, children in the intervention group demonstrated greater improvement in teacher-rated prosocial behavior and emotion regulation than children in the control group. They also received better grades at the end of the school year. In addition, over the course of the intervention, children in the control group demonstrated an increase in ego-centric behavior, as measured by a behavioral task, while children who received the Kindness Curriculum did not.

Music training

Music training is another powerful health-promoting activity for children.[25] As have studies of contemplative interventions, most studies of music interventions have focused on older children and adolescents. The overwhelming majority of these studies also have been conducted with children with specific health conditions. Two literature reviews have summarized the results of randomized controlled trials (RCTs) of music-based interventions.

Mrázová and Celec[26] presented results of 28 RCTs of music interventions with children and adolescents, conducted mostly with children with serious health conditions. Twenty-three of the 28 studies (82%) indicated significant positive effects of the interventions on mostly socioemotional outcomes (eg, pain, procedure-related distress, anxiety, and depressive symptoms). The interventions varied widely in length and format, making it difficult to draw firm conclusions about their active therapeutic features.

Another review of RCTs was conducted by Naylor and colleagues,[27] who summarized results of 17 RCTs (only 5 of which were also reviewed by Mrázová and Celec[26]). Across the 17 trials, the effects of music interventions were mixed, yielding both positive and null findings for a wide range of socioemotional outcomes. The review included 4 studies conducted with mostly young children. In all 4, music interventions yielded significant improvements for most key outcome variables, such as reaching developmental milestones (children with developmental delays), social skills (children with autism), coping with illness (children with cancer), and enjoyment (children with cystic fibrosis).

Standley[28] conducted a meta-analysis of 30 studies that tested the effect of music interventions on the reading competency for children attending preschool through junior high school. The effect of music interventions on children's reading was small, but significant (Cohen $d = 0.32$). It was not uniform across children's ages, ranging from large ($d = 0.62$), to small ($d = 0.25$), to null ($d = 0.00$) for pre-kindergarten, elementary school, and junior high, respectively.

Although the literature on the health promoting effects of enrichment activities in early childhood is ironically in its infancy, it indicates that enrichment activities, such as yoga, mindfulness, and music training, are associated with a range of emotional and behavioral health and academic outcomes for young children. Children may even benefit from the contemplative interventions that are offered only to their parents.[23]

The health-promoting enrichment activities, including yoga, mindfulness, and music training, are another essential component of the VFBA. The VFBA family health programs often begin with the FWCs helping families to make arrangements for the enrichment activities for children. These enjoyable and nonthreatening activities offer FWCs a comfortable context to build a relationship with the family. In addition to their direct effects on the health and well being of family members, the enrichment activities thus help to engage families in the VFBA program.

SUMMARY

Our literature review indicated that parents of young children can benefit from receiving coaching in health-promoting family routines and practices, such as healthy bedtime routines or parenting techniques that minimize screen time. Parents of young children also can benefit from coaching in positive parenting skills. The review also indicated that significant emotional and behavioral problems challenge the parents' ability to provide health-promoting family routines and their effective discipline practices, ultimately threatening successful child development. There is also growing empirical evidence indicating that enrichment activities have health-promoting effects for children. Because music training appears to have the strongest impact on children's development during the early childhood period, it would be reasonable to expect that for other enrichment activities as well.

Informed by these findings, the VFBA offers evidence-based health promotion, prevention, and intervention to the entire family. This means that both children and parents receive direct assessment, health promotion, prevention, and, where indicated, intervention. The VFBA built on a premise that all parents can benefit from support in providing health-promoting family routines and practices and in using positive parenting skills. This is especially true for families in which parents are experiencing significant emotional and behavioral problems that challenge effective parenting. The VFBA also emphasizes health-promoting enrichment activities, both because of their positive effects on family health and their utility in engaging families in the VFBA program.

ARTICLE SUMMARY

- All health is tied to emotional behavioral health.
- The family is an influential health-promoting social institution. Families promote health through daily routines and practices.
- Parents can be coached to create health-promoting family routines and practices and to use positive parenting strategies.
- Parental emotional and behavioral problems impair the parents' ability to provide health-promoting family routines and practices and to use effective parenting strategies, which ultimately negatively affects their children's health. Healthcare efforts supporting children should thus directly address parental emotional and behavioral health.
- Enrichment activities, such as contemplative practices and music training, are gaining empirical support for promoting children's health.
- The VFBA is a public health paradigm that emphasizes emotional and behavioral health, focuses on the entire family, and uses individualized, evidence-based health promotion, prevention, and intervention.
- VFBA assessment includes assessment of each family member's emotional and behavioral and general health, family routines and practices, parenting, enrichment activities, and family relationships. Both children and parents are directly assessed.
- As part of the VFBA, each family is partnered with an FWC, who helps parents to develop and implement a comprehensive plan of health and wellness, including health-promoting family routines and practices and positive parenting skills. The FWC also helps family members to engage in evidence-based enrichment activities.
- Where indicated by the results of family based assessment, families are also partnered with an FFC, a family based, evidence-based psychotherapist, and with a family based psychiatrist.

REFERENCES

1. Prince M, Patel V, Saxena S, et al. No health without mental health. Lancet 2007; 370(9590):859–77.
2. Salovey P, Rothman A, Detweiler JB, et al. Emotional states and physical health. Am Psychol 2000;55:110–21.
3. Cohen S, Pressman SD. Positive affect and health. Curr Dir Psychol Sci 2006;15: 122–5.
4. Hudziak JJ, Bartels M. Genetic and environmental influences on wellness, resilience, and psychopathology: a family based approach for promotion, prevention, and intervention. In: Hudziak JJ, editor. Psychopathology and wellness: genetic and environmental influences. Arlington (VA): American Psychiatric Publishing; 2008. p. 267–86.
5. Denham SA. Relationships between family rituals, family routines, and health. J Fam Nurs 2003;9(3):305–30.
6. Christensen P. The health-promoting family: a conceptual framework for future research. Soc Sci Med 2004;59(2):377–87.

7. Ivanova M. Family assessment and feedback intervention: a training manual. Burlington (VT): University of Vermont Department of Psychiatry; 2014.
8. Mindell JA, Kuhn B, Lewin DS, et al. Behavioral treatment of bedtime problems and night wakings in infants and young children. Sleep 2006;29(10): 1263–76.
9. Schmidt ME, Haines J, O'Brien A, et al. Systematic review of effective strategies for reducing screen time among young children. Obesity 2012;20(7): 1338–54.
10. McMahon RJ, Forehand RL. Helping the noncompliant child: family-based treatment for oppositional behavior. 2nd edition. New York: Guilford Press; 2015.
11. Webster-Stratton C. The incredible years: a trouble shooting guide for parents of children ages 2-8. Seattle (WA): Incredible Years; 2006.
12. Kazdin AE. Parent management training: treatment for oppositional, aggressive, and antisocial behavior in children and adolescents. New York: Oxford University Press; 2005.
13. Sanders MR, Markie-Dadds C, Turner KMT. Practitioner's manual for standard triple P. Brisbane (Australia): Families International Publishing; 2000.
14. Maughan DR, Christiansen E, Jenson WR, et al. Behavioral parent training as a treatment for externalizing behaviors and disruptive behavior disorders: a meta-analysis. Sch Psychol Rev 2005;34(3):267–86.
15. Lundahl B, Risser HJ, Lovejoy MC. A meta-analysis of parent training: moderators and follow-up effects. Clin Psychol Rev 2006;26:86–104.
16. Dishion TJ, Shaw D, Connell A, et al. The family check-up with high-risk indigent families: preventing problem behavior by increasing parents' positive behavior support in early childhood. Child Dev 2008;79(5):1395–414.
17. Dishion TJ, Stormshak EA. Intervening in children's lives: an ecological, family-centered approach to mental health care. Washington, DC: American Psychological Association; 2007.
18. Dishion TJ, Brennan LM, Shaw DS, et al. Prevention of problem behavior through annual family check-ups in early childhood: intervention effects from home to early elementary school. J Abnorm Child Psychol 2014;42(3):343–54.
19. Berg-Nielsen T, Vikan A, Dahl AA. Parenting related to child and parental psychopathology: a descriptive review of the literature. Clin Child Psychol Psychiatry 2002;7(4):529–52.
20. Zajicek-Farber M, Mayer LM, Daughtery LG. Connections among parental mental health, stress, child routines, and early emotional behavioral regulation of preschool children in low-income families. J Soc Social Work Res 2012;3(1): 31–50.
21. Hur E, Buettner CK, Jeon L. Parental depressive symptoms and children's school-readiness: the indirect effect of household chaos. J Child Fam Stud 2015;24(11): 3462–73.
22. Greenberg MT, Harris AR. Nurturing mindfulness in children and youth: current state of research. Child Dev Perspect 2012;6(2):161–6.
23. Fisak B. The prevention of anxiety in preschool-aged children: development of a new program and preliminary findings. Ment Health Prev 2014;2:18–25.
24. Flook L, Goldberg SB, Pinger L, et al. Promoting prosocial behavior and self-regulatory skills in preschool children through a mindfulness-based kindness curriculum. Dev Psychol 2015;51(1):44–51.
25. Hudziak JJ, Albaugh MD, Ducharme S, et al. Cortical thickness maturation and duration of music training: health-promoting activities shape brain development. J Am Acad Child Adolesc Psychiatry 2014;53(11):1153–61.

26. Mrázová M, Celec P. A systematic review of randomized controlled trials using music therapy for children. J Altern Complement Med 2010;16(10): 1089–95.

27. Naylor KT, Kingsnorth S, Lamont A, et al. The effectiveness of music in pediatric healthcare: a systematic review of randomized controlled trials. Evid Based Complement Alternat Med 2011;2011:464759.

28. Standley JM. Does music instruction help children learn to read? Evidence of a meta-analysis. App Res Music Educ 2008;27(1):17–32.

The Neurobiological Impact of Postpartum Maternal Depression

Prevention and Intervention Approaches

Stacy S. Drury, MD, PhD[a],*, Laura Scaramella, PhD[b], Charles H. Zeanah, MD[a]

KEYWORDS

- Postpartum depression • Psychotherapy • Dyadic interventions • Neurobiology
- Early life stress • Infants

KEY POINTS

- Postpartum depression (PPD) is a highly prevalent public health concern with implications for infant neurobiological outcomes.
- To date, evidence for universal and selected interventions is limited in terms of efficacy for the treatment of PPD, and there is a dearth of evidence for the impact of any intervention on infant neurodevelopmental outcomes.
- A small but growing body of research suggests that indicated psychotherapeutic interventions have positive effects on infant neurobiological outcomes.
- Greater incorporation of biological outcomes in both infants and mothers is needed to improve long-term infant and maternal outcomes in women at risk for PPD.

INTRODUCTION

PPD represents a significant public health problem with prevalence estimates ranging from 12% to 19% and clear negative implications for both maternal and infant health and wellness.[1–3] Although risk factors for PPD are generally similar to those for depression at other time points in the life course, the substantial neuroendocrine changes that occur in a mother immediately after birth and the significant increase in contextual stressors that accompany caring for an infant may compound these

Disclosures: The authors report no commercial or financial disclosures.
a Department of Psychiatry and Behavioral Sciences, Tulane University, 1430 Tulane avenue, #8055, New Orleans, LA 70112, USA; b Department of Psychology, The University of New Orleans, 2000 Lakeshore Drive, New Orleans, LA 70148, USA
* Corresponding author. Department of Psychiatry and Behavioral Sciences, Tulane University, 1430 Tulane Avenue, #8055, New Orleans, LA 70112.
E-mail address: sdrury@tulane.edu

risks.[3–6] For instance, using data from the National Epidemiologic Survey on Alcohol and Related Conditions, Le Strat and colleagues[7] compared characteristics of women currently or within the past year pregnant with and without depression. Demographically, depressed women were more likely to be unmarried, multipara, and ethnic minority status. Compared with nondepressed women, depressed mothers also were more likely to be under the age of 25, have lower income levels, and be less educated. Depressed mothers were significantly more likely to use illicit substances and were 8 times more likely to also suffer from other psychiatric disorders than nondepressed women or nondepressed mothers.[8] Repeatedly, risk for PPD has been linked to increased exposure to stressful life events.[7] Demographic stressors, like teenage parenthood[9] or military involvement (eg, military wives),[10] have also been associated with elevated PPD. Exposure to both early life adversity as well as current life stressors, such as unemployment, change in marital status, death of a loved one, and disease, seems to increase risk for PPD, particularly among women with presumed genetic vulnerability and with limited access to protective resources (eg, social support and financial support).[11] Unfortunately, these same risk factors may affect maternal caregiving, potentially resulting in a synergistic negative effect on infant neurobiological development.

Given the significant number of maternal-infant dyads affected by PPD, there is a growing interest in developing better population-wide and demographically focused efforts to increase PPD identification and implement effective treatment. Public health approaches to preventive interventions distinguish among universal, selective, and indicated interventions.[12] Universal interventions include health promotion efforts and intervention efforts aimed at a broad population. Public service messages addressing PPD, for example, might help women recognize how PPD differs from more typical symptoms of exhaustion, sleep disruption, and emotional lability that are prevalent in the weeks after delivery of a child. Selective interventions target members of a group who have high lifetime or high imminent risk for depression. Some estimates indicate that almost 40% of women with children under the age of 3 years old and who live in stressful urban environments, for example, have elevated levels of depressive symptoms.[13] An intervention to prevent depression that targets impoverished, inner-city mothers after the birth of a child is a selective intervention. Finally, indicated preventions target those who manifest depressive symptoms that may later become a full-blown disorder. Referral of women who screen positive on the Edinburgh Postnatal Depression Scale,[14] or a similar measure, at the 6-week postpartum check-up in a perinatal intervention program is an indicated intervention.

Particularly for pediatric health care providers, including mental health, the public health relevance of PPD extends beyond mothers to include the effects of both the illness itself and intervention efforts on their infants. With this in mind, preventive interventions can also be evaluated in their ability to buffer the impact of maternal depression on her offspring. Despite the clear links between maternal PPD and negative child outcomes, the impact of current efforts targeting the prevention and/or treatment of PPD to also diminish the negative impact on child outcomes remains limited. In older children, evidence of the positive effects of treatment of parental depression for both children and parents has been reported, although for the most part this has been limited to examination of the effects on child psychopathology without exploration of other health and biological outcomes.[15,16] For young children, where maternal depression is more likely to substantially influence caregiving and the dyadic relationship, the few existing studies that have explored the direct impact of PPD interventions on infant short-term and long-term outcomes suggest that current approaches are insufficient to protect or buffer offspring from the harmful effects of PPD.[17]

This review focuses on infant neurodevelopmental outcomes associated specifically with PPD and its treatment. The neurodevelopmental and health effects of medication use, specifically selective serotonin reuptake inhibitors, on prenatally exposed infants remain a highly prolific area of research covered in depth elsewhere and are beyond the scope of this review (for reviews, see Refs.[18–20]). In examining the impact of interventions on neurobiological outcomes in offspring, the authors propose that a focus consistent with the Research Domain Criteria[21] on neural systems and biological pathways, as opposed to diagnostic categories, provides greater insight into needed next research steps. Despite established links between PPD and myriad negative health outcomes across the life course, the mechanisms and specific pathways through which this elevated risk is embedded remain poorly defined. Disentangling mechanisms and moderators that include shared and independent genetic liability; familial environment, such as social support, paternal factors, and parental discord; infant temperament; and other factors is a needed, albeit complex, next step with significant public health and policy implications. Delineating the modifiable factors, aspects of preexisting risk, and specific treatment components associated with improved child outcomes, is expected to enhance the efficacy of PPD interventions, not only for reducing maternal symptoms but also for promoting infant health and development. Given the challenge, particularly in young children, of eliciting data about psychological symptoms from sources other than caregivers, and the potential impact of depression symptoms on parent report of child behavior, establishing biomarkers of both vulnerability and resilience in infants exposed to maternal PPD is critical. The pressing need for these advances is further highlighted by the existing literature, albeit limited, suggesting that treatment of maternal depression does not necessarily result in improved maternal-child interactions, one of the key proposed mechanisms through which PPD has a negative impact on infant outcomes.[22]

Infant Neurodevelopment

The intricate development of the human brain begins only a few short weeks after conception and continues for decades. During the first years of life, there is tremendous overgrowth and differentiation of the neural substrate. Multiple processes are involved in this initial period of rapid brain growth, including cellular migration, neurogenesis, dendritic branching, and axonal formation. It is on this basic early architecture of the brain that subsequent neurodevelopment and function depends. After an initial overgrowth and proliferation, the shaping and refining of neural circuits through synaptogenesis, apoptosis, and myelination occur in an experience-dependent manner. That is, synapses that are stimulated repeatedly tend to strengthen, creating consolidated circuits that are then myelinated. Synapses that do not receive repeated stimulation are lost, a process called pruning, which subsequently results in apoptosis, or programmed cellular death. The rate by which the refining of these neural circuits occurs differs throughout the brain, with protracted refinement in some areas, such as the prefrontal cortex, well into adolescence and early adulthood. The refining of these circuits is directly influenced by experience and, particularly during infancy and early childhood, is intricately linked to a young child's experience of caregiving.

The impact of maternal care on neurodevelopmental processes is an area of active research, both in terms of understanding the consequences of appropriate, contingent, and sensitive caregiving and in relation to defining the lasting negative consequences of atypical caregiving, including the effects of maternal depression.[3,16,23–26] Mothers, both in humans and across mammalian species, serve as potent external regulators of infant neurodevelopment, physiology, and emotion regulation.[27–31] As such, variations or deviations in the expected caregiving experience, such as often occurs with PPD, are expected to influence an infant's developing neurobiological processes, likely resulting in lifelong alterations.

Postpartum Depression and the Spectrum of Postpartum Disorders

The emergence of PPD may begin with the appearance of the postpartum blues. Postpartum blues typically occurs during the first 2 weeks of childbirth, with the strongest link to the physiologic drop in levels of circulating hormones and massive diuresis after delivery. Symptoms are generally short lived and include crying, confusion, mood lability, anxiety, and sadness.[4] No demographic or cultural factors have been demonstrated to significantly increase risk for postpartum blues.[32] Currently, no available evidence links postpartum blues not escalating to PPD to any adverse effects on children. Given that postpartum blues on its own is fleeting and minor in impairment, the condition is not the focus of subsequent discussion. Its chief importance is that approximately 20% of women who experience postpartum blues subsequently develop PPD; as such, postpartum blues represents an important risk factor.[33] An alternative perspective, to date unexplored, is that an enhanced understanding of the 80% of women who do not develop PPD may provide novel insight into preventive approaches.

Differing from postpartum blues, PPD symptoms match those of a major depressive episode and include sadness, loss of interest in previously pleasurable activities, sleep disturbance, loss of energy, weight changes, concentration problems, agitation, feelings of worthlessness or guilt, or thoughts of suicide and meet similar duration and intensity criteria to typical depression.[34] In rare cases, new mothers exhibit a severe, postpartum disorder known as postpartum psychosis, involving delusions, hallucinations, and gross functional impairment.[35] Postpartum psychosis typically appears during the first 3 months after childbirth.[4] Symptoms are often consistent with a bipolar disorder.[36] Postpartum psychosis represents the rarest form of the major 3 postpartum disorders, with an incidence rate of 1 to 2 cases per 1000 births.[37]

Neurodevelopmental Impact of Maternal Postpartum Depression

The impact of PPD crosses multiple domains for both mothers and infants.[3,26,38] In addition to health impacts, the impact of maternal depression has also been evaluated in terms of its economic impact in relation to elevated health care utilization as well as other costs, such as lost wages, increased costs associated with special education, and so forth—factors of heightened relevance in the current economic climate.[39,40] Negative effects of PPD on offspring include increased risk of insecure attachment and poorer cognitive, language, social-emotional, and behavioral development.[26,41] In smaller prospective studies and larger epidemiologic samples, PPD has been associated with increased risk for internalizing symptoms at 18 months of age as well as increased rates of internalizing disorders throughout childhood and adolescence.[42–45] Elevated rates of externalizing symptoms, including physical aggression, also have been reported across childhood, suggesting that PPD has an impact on multiple neural pathways.[2,46–48] Other neurobiological consequences of PPD have been reported, including decreased diurnal cortisol, altered stress cortisol reactivity, inattention, social disengagement, lower IQ, and language delays.[49–54] Infants of mothers with PPD are reported to exhibit less positive facial and vocal expressions and be more irritable and avoidant.[55] Additionally, there is evidence of the association between PPD and poor infant physical growth across the first year of life, an effect that was stronger than socioeconomic status and remained even after controlling for infant birth weight.[56] Although much of the work summarized in this article reflects findings specific to PPD, distinguishing between the effects of prenatal and postnatal exposure and the delineation of moderating and mediating pathways is challenging.[26,57,58]

The relation between maternal depression and infant negative outcomes has been explained, in part, by the impact of depression on maternal interactional behaviors and distorted maternal cognitions about her infant and about parenting.[59] Meta-analyses of studies reporting on the impact of maternal depression on maternal behavior note that depressed mothers are more irritable and/or hostile, less engaged with their infants, play less with their infants, and demonstrate decreased positive emotion and warmth.[60,61] Depressed mothers also may be more aggressive in their parenting strategies and less emotionally responsive to their offspring. Infants and toddlers of mothers with depression have been found to exhibit increased rates of insecure attachment, reduced social engagement, increased negativity, and poor fear regulation.[43,50,62,63] One interesting unanswered question is whether maternal difficulties in establishing relationships with infants, or a diminished positive experience of the relationship, is reflective of the underlying neurobiology of depression or a preexisting risk factor that contributes to the development of PPD.[22]

PPD also influences other caregiving and health related practices, which independently may effect neurobiological development, suggesting innovative targets for universal, targeted, and selected interventions.[64] At the extreme, studies have examined the impact of maternal depression on early childhood neglect and aggression/discipline.[65] Depressed mothers are more likely than their nondepressed counterparts to engage in neglectful behaviors, such as leaving children home alone.[66–68] Depressed mothers also are more likely to report being irritable,[69] having increased negative emotions, feeling less invested, and using more physical discipline with their children than nondepressed mothers.[70–73]

In addition to elevated risk of abuse and neglect, mothers with PPD are more likely to engage in less optimal feeding practices, including decreased rates of breastfeeding; increased rates of inappropriate feeding habits, like introducing cereal and juice earlier than recommended; and decreased rates of well-child visits and fewer vaccinations.[74] Mothers with PPD have decreased rates of reading, playing, and talking with infants as well as less adherence to daily routines.[64,75] The impact of PPD on these other aspects of caregiving may play a role in infant neurodevelopmental disruptions. For instance, lower rates of reading to children may influence the development of language deficits associated with PPD, a model that has yet to be examined.[75] Despite the likelihood that these other dimensions of caregiving can compound the negative impact of PPD, traditional psychotherapy and/or pharmacotherapy does not routinely address them. Although it seems intuitive that effective treatment of maternal depressive symptoms is needed to prevent or ameliorate the negative effects on offspring, this remains to be empirically tested in well-designed studies and, in part, would rely on data defining the mechanisms through which PPD results in negative neurobiological outcomes.[2,76]

UNIVERSAL, SELECTED, AND INDICATED EFFORTS FOR MATERNAL POSTPARTUM DEPRESSION

The ideal goal of all public health efforts centers on prevention. In the case of the lasting impact of PPD on infant neurodevelopment, prevention efforts may serve to prevent both maternal depression and the negative effects on infant neurodevelopment and health. Given evidence supporting the intergenerational risk of depression,[77,78] particularly associated with early childhood abuse,[79,80] prevention efforts focused on enhancing maternal sensitivity and contingent caregiving among mothers with a history of child abuse, a substantial risk factor for both PPD and caregiving deficits regardless of their own depressive status, may provide an innovative approach to intergenerational protection. The next section discusses nonpharmacologic treatment of PPD, providing a broad overview of the efficacy of universal, targeted, and indicated efforts on PPD, with specific attention to the few studies that have examined the impact of these interventions on infant outcomes. Strengths and weaknesses of data are identified at each level as well as the gaps in the research. Lastly, a targeted research agenda is proposed that leverages evidence for best approaches and novel biological indicators suggested that may provide enhanced evidence of the efficacy of these approaches.

Universal

Universal efforts focus on health promotion and/or efforts aimed at a broad population. One of the primary approaches for PPD has been the implementation of universal screening of mothers for PPD by a variety of health care providers, including obstetricians, pediatricians, nurses, lactation consultants, birthing centers, and Women, Infants and Children (WIC) agencies that are the most likely care providers for screening for PPD. The World Health Organization, American Academy of Pediatrics, and American College of Obstetricians and Gynecologists recommend universal screening at all postpartum and well-child visits.[1,81,82] To be effective, universal screening must be both practical and accurate. Studies have examined the utility of a range of different screenings, very brief (eg, 2 or 3 questions) and longer question screens, finding that both short screens and longer screens are effective in identifying PPD, particularly within the primary care setting.[83] Although the implementation of universal screening within primary care settings has resulted in significant increased PPD identification and referrals,[81] to date the impact of these screening on actual maternal depression levels is equivocal,[84] and the downstream effect on neurobiological outcomes in offspring has yet to be studied.

Universal screening

In May 2015, the American College of Obstetricians and Gynecologists released a committee opinion regarding screening for perinatal depression. This report noted that PPD symptoms often go under-recognized and under-reported due to the failure of both providers and mothers to differentiate between normal physiologic changes and pathologic symptoms.[1,85] The consequences of perinatal maternal depression for infant development is pervasive, prompting efforts to improve screening and treatment efforts, including the American College of Obstetricians and Gynecologists recommendations for implementation of systems to ensure follow-up for diagnosis and treatment are needed.[1] Screening efforts using a variety of established measures (Center for Epidemiologic Studies Depression Scale, Edinburgh Postnatal Depression Scale, and Beck Depression Inventory) have been found to successfully identify major and minor depression during pregnancy and offer established and simple measures to incorporate within routine prenatal care for medical providers, including obstetricians and pediatricians.[83] Screening tools are generally more accurate in detecting major depression compared with minor depression.[84] Despite the established risks associated with PPD and the availability of practical screening measures, the use of validated tools to identify PPD is rare in obstetric practices. Overall screening rates often fall below 50% and the percentage of mothers actually entering treatment, once identified, is even lower.[83,86,87] When considering a targeted goal of ameliorating the negative neurobiological impact of PPD on offspring, an alternative venue in which to implement universal screening is a well-child visits, particularly because pediatricians may be the only medical providers routinely encountered by mothers during a child's first years of life.[81] Similar to screening within obstetrics, the need for rapid, practical screens and referral options is critical to effective universal efforts at this level.[88]

Universal interventions

In addition to universal screening, universal prevention efforts have been explored. Interventions include educational, peer support, massage, group support, and structured psychotherapies. The effectiveness of these interventions, however, varies. Analyses suggest that universal preventive efforts have not been cost effective and are significantly less effective than targeted or indicated efforts.[89–93] To date, few of these have evaluated the impact of preventive interventions on infant neurobiological outcomes. Evidence of the positive impact on infants of universal interventions targeting anticipatory guidance about breastfeeding, playing, sleep, book reading/talking, and nutrition have been reported. Unfortunately, examination of the impact on maternal mood in these studies is absent. Universal intervention studies that focus on parental behaviors known to be impacted by predisposing factors associated with PPD (eg, previous depressive episode, age, and child maltreatment) that concurrently measure the impact on both maternal mood and infant neurobiological development are needed.

A variety of different universal home-visiting and community support intervention programs have been studied, with varying levels of scientific rigor. In a randomized study examining both the impact and cost-effectiveness of community in-home support on PPD, no evidence of effectiveness was found.[92] Data combined with other studies suggested that universal home-visiting programs are neither effective nor cost effective and instead interventions targeting specific, at-risk populations are needed and have demonstrated efficacy (discussed later).[94–97] In a low-risk, universal home-visiting intervention, women who had low levels of depression symptoms at 6 weeks postpartum showed significant reductions in depressed mood, suggesting a stronger protective effect of these interventions among low-risk mothers.[98]

Cognitive behavior therapy (CBT) is an intervention for both the treatment and prevention of depression. A recent meta-analysis examined studies of CBT for treatment and prevention of perinatal depression, including PPD.[99] Although CBT demonstrated some evidence of efficacy for maternal depressive symptoms when administered at the community level, its impact was small when administered prenatally. Greatest evidence of efficacy for PPD was found when CBT was provided to highest-risk individuals, administered postnatally, and provided as individual therapy as opposed to group therapy.[99] The impact of CBT on infant neurobiological outcomes, however, remains unknown.

In conclusion, despite widespread recognition of both the frequency and the negative impact of PPD, current approaches to implementing both universal screening and universal prevention efforts have demonstrated only minimal impact on maternal outcomes.[89,100] Well-designed studies of universal interventions have not yet evaluated the impact on infant neurodevelopment. With this body of evidence in mind, efforts to decrease the negative impact of PPD on infant outcomes likely need to be either selected or indicated as efficacious.

Selected

Selected interventions require identification of individuals at heightened risk. In cases of PPD, the risks are, in general, similar to those for major depression and include previous history of depression, elevated financial stress and strain (eg, unemployed status, financial hardship, and poverty), heightened marital stress and strain (eg, marital conflict, separation, and divorce), diminished social support, and a family history of depression.[5,6,101,102] Moreover, women reporting low socioeconomic status, defined as a combination of having low income, having less than a college education, being unmarried, and being unemployed, were at an 11-fold greater risk for postnatal depression compared with women reporting high socioeconomic status.[6] Strong evidence indicates that women with history of neglect, sexual abuse, and other early traumatic life events are at particular risk for perinatal depression, a risk moderated by both current life stressors and potentially maternal race.[5,103,104] This relationship between elevated risk of PPD in women with a history of child maltreatment may be compounded because maltreatment is also associated with altered immunologic and neuroendocrine regulation, factors that are independently linked to both poor birth outcomes and PPD.[105,106] Increased risk for PPD is associated with preterm delivery and infant care in the neonatal intensive care unit (NICU). Exposure to abuse during childhood is a risk factor for maternal depression during the perinatal period, and subsequently maternal depression in the perinatal period is associated with elevated risk of both child maltreatment and depression in her offspring.[107,108] This cyclic and intergenerational impact suggests that careful assessment of the effects of child maltreatment on maternal neurobiology and mothering behavior, irrespective of depressive status, might identify mechanistic pathways contributing to multigenerational risk for depression. Evidence is accumulating to suggest that pregnant women and mothers of young children should be screened for history of childhood abuse and offered interventions to improve their own well-being, ideally preventing serious long-term health disparities in their offspring and potentially subsequent generations as well.

One targeted population with significantly elevated rates of PPD is mothers whose infants are in the NICU. Rates of PPD are substantially higher among mothers of children in the NICU, as are rates of posttraumatic stress disorder and other anxiety disorders.[109] Although recognizing the need for enhanced identification of PPD in the NICU, to date it is unclear who are the best providers to implement this screening.[110] Targeted interventions may decrease PPD among these mothers, with some, but not all, interventions demonstrating moderate efficacy.[111–114] Infant outcomes positively impacted by these interventions include increased rates of secure attachment,[115] improved feeding behaviors,[112] decreased irritability and colic,[116] and enhanced cognitive functioning at 2 years of age.[117] Additionally, although other attachment and dyadic focused interventions have demonstrated efficacy in improving infant neurobiological outcomes with preterm babies,[118,119] these interventions did not assess the impact on maternal mood, despite evidence that disrupted maternal-infant relationships are related to PPD risk. Future studies to examine potential bidirectional effects are warranted.

Selected interventions

In a recent review of PPD preventive interventions by Werner and colleagues, of the 37 randomized controlled trials, only 17 were found effective, and of these 13 were targeted to at-risk populations, supporting the hypothesis that the greatest efficacy for prevention is associated with selected populations. Several important barriers to these interventions have been proposed, including inconsistent measurement of PPD and high rates of attrition, potentially as consequences of stigma, accessibility, and a sole focus on the mother.[93,120] Feasibility of Web-based and smartphone-based interventions for PPD to address accessibility challenges have been piloted and represent innovative future directions.[121–125] Examples of larger selected interventions targeting depression after the first year of life have found that improvement in maternal depression symptoms mediated the effect of family-based treatment on toddlers externalizing and internalizing symptoms; however, this was not specific to PPD.[126]

Despite evidence that universal CBT was, for the most part, ineffective in decreasing PPD risk, CBT provided to selected high-risk populations seems to have some efficacy in decreasing depression risk as well as in mood regulation and coping, factors expected to have direct implications for maternal caregiving.[3,127–129] The effects in the majority of studies are modest, however, likely due to high rates of attrition and flaws in study design.[3] Feasibility trials of cognitive behavioral–based online interventions for at-risk mothers may result in greater efficacy given that accessibility of treatment has been identified as a primary barrier to effective selected interventions.[123,130] In at least 1 study, CBT has demonstrated unique effects on infant neurobiological outcomes, specifically cortisol levels.[128] In this study, high-risk mothers, defined by past history of depression or elevated depressive symptoms during the second trimester, were randomized to CBT or usual treatment. A positive effect on both maternal and infant cortisol levels was detected at 6 months postpartum, suggesting a joint neurobiological effect.[128]

Home-based interventions for at-risk mothers have been evaluated, and although several studies have demonstrated positive effects on depression, this has not been universal.[131] Unexpectedly, a study of low-income mothers who received a home-based, peer support intervention with education about maternal-infant interactions found that the control group demonstrated greater reductions in depressive symptoms and better maternal-infant interactions, the opposite of expected outcomes. The investigators ascribe these discrepant results to the use of peer, rather than professional, home visitors. No impact on infant IQ or salivary cortisol was detected.[132] In a tiered home-visiting program, with specialty-trained home visitors, home visiting seemed protective against PPD through 18 months of age; however, the impact of this intervention on infant outcomes was not evaluated.[133] The preventive impact of telephone-based peer mentoring for at-risk mothers has also been explored. Although efficacy of decreasing depressive risk was reported, to date the impact on infant outcomes has not been reported.[90] Fussy Babies, a tiered individualized intervention,[134] has demonstrated positive effects on maternal well-being, depression, and parenting stress among women who received the intervention compared with waiting list controls; however, to date, the impact on infant neurobiological or health outcomes has not been evaluated.

Although a significant number of psychotherapeutic and educational approaches have been studied as selected interventions for PPD, alternative interventions targeting infant behavior or caregiving factors associated with elevated PPD risk also have been proposed. Infant sleep problems, for example, seem to have a bidirectional relationship with maternal PPD, with evidence of poor sleep practices among mothers with PPD as well as elevated risk of PPD among mothers with infants experiencing sleep problems.[135,136] Furthermore, infant sleep problems are independently associated with poor maternal-infant attachment, less sophisticated child cognitive development, and elevated risk of child maltreatment.[137] Several randomized trials have examined the impact of sleep interventions on both maternal mood and child developmental outcomes, demonstrating consistent evidence of a positive effect on maternal mood, child sleep, and child behavior problems.[135,138,139] The long-term neurobiological and health effects of these interventions beyond the toddler years has yet to be examined. Despite the evidence of efficacy of infant sleep strategies, to date this has not been integrated into other indicated or selected interventions for PPD. Another small pilot study examined the impact of problem-solving education on low-income mothers of preterm infants, finding decreased rates of PPD, but this study failed to concurrently explore infant outcomes.[111]

In conclusion, selected interventions have demonstrated modest efficacy in decreasing PPD in selected, high-risk, populations. To date, there is insufficient evidence to suggest that one type of intervention is more efficacious than another in preventing PPD. Intuitively, dyadic-based interventions might be expected to demonstrate enhanced positive effects on infant outcomes compared with interventions specifically targeting mothers; however, this has yet to be empirically tested. Few studies have examined the impact of selected interventions on infant outcomes, an area much in need of research. Based on the existing, albeit limited, data, it seems that CBT selected interventions show promise for neurobiological effects on infants and mothers.[128,132] The positive findings associated with sleep interventions suggest that integration of sleep education and support into other interventions may have particular utility. Given the growing evidence of efficacy for selected interventions on maternal depression, there is a clear need to evaluate the short-term and long-term impact on both maternal and infant neurobiological outcomes. Future research that focuses on selected interventions targeting maternal biological markers of elevated PPD depression risk, including genetic liability or neuroendocrine markers, is an innovative and needed next research step, particularly because genetic and neurobiological markers may have shared influences on both mother and infant.[140,141]

Indicated

The established links between PPD and negative infant outcomes suggest that treatment of PPD should result in improvement in maternal-infant interactions and infant behavior, health, and neurobiology. In contrast to the wide variability in efficacy for universal and selected interventions, indicated nonpharmacologic interventions for PPD have demonstrated modest efficacy in decreasing maternal depressive symptoms.[142] These interventions include support groups, home visiting, peer volunteer telephone support, CBT, psychodynamic therapy, and interpersonal therapy (IPT).[3,17,22,143–145] Therapeutic interventions for PPD also differ widely on their focus relative to the infant and the mother-child relationship, with some only including the mother and some specifically focusing on the dyad.

A meta-analysis of the impact of psychotherapy for maternal depression on child outcomes identified 9 studies that met inclusion, with 5 of these studies focused on PPD and young children.[146] Overall, positive effects on both infant behavior and maternal-infant interactions were detected. CBT and IPT were not significantly different from each other in terms of infant outcomes, consistent with an earlier comprehensive review that found that treatment of PPD resulted in improved maternal-infant interactions as reported by mothers.[22] Few of these studies examined the impact of maternal treatment on direct measures of infant cognition, behavior, and health, as opposed to maternal report, a potential confound that warrants future study.[22]

Maternal psychotherapeutic interventions

IPT is an established treatment of depression, including PPD, in both individual and group settings.[17,147,148] Although IPT decreased parenting stress, at least 1 study did not find improvement in maternal report of infant attachment, behavior, or temperament, suggesting that IPT alone is not sufficient to protect infants from the negative impact of PPD.[17] A more recent study of IPT found effectiveness not only for maternal symptoms but also mother-infant interactions assessed through trained observers.[149] Similar to the effect of toddler-parent psychotherapy, genetic factors seem to moderate maternal response to IPT.[150] An intriguing future direction of research might be to explore whether infant genotype moderates the impact of PPD treatment on infant outcomes.

CBT also has significant evidence to support its use to treat maternal depression, including PPD. Improvement in infant cognitive outcomes has been demonstrated after treatment of PPD in several, but not all, studies that evaluated CBT and other therapies.[144,151,152] In a randomized controlled trial comparing CBT, nondirective supportive therapy, and psychodynamic therapy with routine primary care for low-risk mothers with PPD, improvement in social emotional and cognitive measures was found in all 3 treatment groups at 18 months of age. These effects did not persist, however, to 5 years of age. The investigators suggest that selecting mothers from a low-risk cohort may account for these findings; selecting higher-risk mothers may have resulted in larger and more persistent findings. The investigators also suggested that for higher-risk women there was not a significant difference between interventions with specialists. From an economic cost-effectiveness perspective, using nondirective supportive therapy may be beneficial. In another randomized trial of group CBT compared to mother-toddler treatment and no treatment groups, no differences in infant outcomes were detected between any randomization arms.[152] Although some evidence of greater decline in child psychological symptoms was suggested in the CBT group, the investigators noted this should be interpreted with caution.

One intervention for prenatal and postnatal anxiety and depression that does not seem to have been studied to date is mindfulness. This is a surprising omission given the increasing number of mindfulness interventions in the field of psychiatry at large. Levels of maternal mindfulness during pregnancy were associated with fewer infant self-regulation problems and less negative affectivity after birth. Although the study focused only on maternal anxiety, this work should be extended to maternal depression and could be applied in universal and selected interventions as well as indicated interventions.[153]

Dyadic interventions

Given the significant evidence that PPD has a negative impact on maternal-infant interactions, several studies have reported on the effectiveness of therapies focused on the maternal-infant relationship, administered both prenatally and postnatally, as well as dyadic therapies.[154] Toddler-parent psychotherapy, provided weekly over the course of a year, has been found to have an impact on attachment classification as well as on IQ in infants of depressed mothers.[145,150,155] The improvement in IQ was limited to verbal IQ and persisted after controlling for covariates. In this study, a significant proportion of the impact was moderated by subsequent maternal depressive episodes, indicating that heightened monitoring and booster sessions ought to be included over the first 5 years of life. Insecure attachment, elevated among mothers with depression, also decreased with toddler-parent psychotherapy. Depressed mothers who received treatment actually demonstrated higher rates of secure attachment than control mothers, hinting that the relationship between PPD and insecure attachment may be bidirectional.[145] Similar to initial risk for PPD, genetic variability seems to have an impact on treatment efficacy, again suggesting that specific women may be more vulnerable to PPD but also more responsive to interventions, as may their offspring.[150]

Child-parent psychotherapy (CPP) is an evidence-based therapy for traumatized mother-child dyads with established effectiveness of maternal functioning in women with a history of complex trauma and/or current exposure to interpersonal violence, factors often associated with maternal depression as well as other psychopathology, such as posttraumatic stress disorder. The improvement in maternal functioning, particularly in relation to her parenting and sensitivity, should have positive effects on infant neurodevelopmental processes. Ideally, effective treatment mitigates the lasting negative consequences of maternal depression. In a more recent study, CPP was administered prenatally to mothers with depression and/or posttraumatic stress disorder. Improvement in mothers' symptoms was strongly correlated with maternal self-report of attachment to their unborn child. Specifically, the greatest improvement in symptoms was found among mothers who, pretreatment, reported less attachment to their infants.[156] This finding is consistent with the attachment-based model on which CPP is based. For mothers with less prenatal attachment, an attachment-derived therapy administered prenatally may significantly improve emerging mother-infant attachment relationships. Evaluation of the impact of this type of intervention on maternal sensitivity, contingent parenting, and dyadic attachment classification in future studies would be useful, as would examinations of neurobiological outcomes in these same infants. A recent pilot randomized controlled trial of Triple P—Positive Parenting Program—in women with PPD found that although Triple P was highly acceptable in women with depression, no significant differences between active treatment and control groups in maternal-infant interactions or depressive symptoms were reported.[157]

Infant massage

Consideration of a range of alternative treatment approaches for PPD is increasing, likely in light of concerns about medication use in pregnancy and breastfeeding and challenges to treatment adherence. Evidence is accumulating to suggest that maternal massage administered prenatally, as well as infant massage postnatally, may not only decrease maternal depressive symptoms but also improve infant neurobiological outcomes.[158–160] In a trial comparing support group to maternal-infant massage for PPD, both groups demonstrated decreased depressive symptoms, but at 1 year postdelivery symptoms were still elevated compared with nondepressed mothers.[158] In nonpregnant studies, massage therapy has been suggested to decrease cortisol and corticotropin and increase oxytocin, although some debate exists.[161,162]

Several individual and dyadic therapies have demonstrated positive effects on postnatal maternal depressive symptoms. Particularly for dyadic interventions, there seem to be positive effects on maternal-infant interactions and beginning support for positive neurobiological effects in infants as well. In light of the limited effectiveness of universal and selected interventions, investment in indicated treatments for PPD, with extended monitoring for recurrence of PPD, is likely the most promising direction for additional research.

SUMMARY

Maternal depression is a pervasive public health problem with substantial economic and health costs mothers and their offspring. Although universal screening efforts seem to increase PPD identification, to date these interventions have been ineffective at reducing PPD and no data exist demonstrating positive downstream impacts on infants. Given this, research focused on defining existing barriers to effective PPD treatment by women identified by universal screening is a high priority. Selected interventions have demonstrated minimal effectiveness on maternal mood symptoms and maternal-infant interactions; unfortunately, there is no evidence of a positive impact on infant neurobiological outcomes, again highlighting needed next research steps. Both dyadic and individual psychotherapies have demonstrated efficacy in the treatment of PPD. A growing body of research indicates that these treatments also improve maternal-infant interactions. There remains a paucity of research, however, exploring the short-term and long-term neurobiological consequences of these interventions on infants. This research gap is somewhat striking given the increasing focus on health and neuroscience across medicine and funding agencies. Studies specifically designed to capture both maternal and infant outcomes are needed. Novel therapies that leverage evidence-based existing dyadic therapies and integrate alternative therapies that address caregiving behaviors influenced by PPD, such as sleep, nutrition, and play, may have synergistic benefits for both mothers and their infants. Efforts to determine shared neurobiological pathways linked to elevated risk for PPD, maternal exposure to child maltreatment, and decreased maternal sensitivity with mothers' own children have the potential to un-cover innovative preventive and therapeutic targets. As burgeoning data suggest that the impact of PPD may span generations, improved efficacy of interventions also may result in lasting effects across future generations.

REFERENCES

1. Committee on Obstetric Practice. American college of obstetricians gynecolo-gists committee opinion no. 630: screening for perinatal depression. Obstet Gynecol 2015;125(5):1268–71.
2. Previti G, Pawlby S, Chowdhury S, et al. Neurodevelopmental outcome for offspring of women treated for antenatal depression: a systematic review. Arch Womens Ment Health 2014;17(6):471–83.
3. O'Hara M, McCabe J. Postpartum depression: current status and future direc-tions. Annu Rev Clin Psychol 2013;9:379–407.
4. Payne J. The role of estrogen in mood disorders in women. Int Rev Psychiatry 2003;15(3):280–90.
5. Meltzer-Brody S, Boschloo L, Jones I, et al. The EPDS-Lifetime: assessment of lifetime prevalence and risk factors for perinatal depression in a large cohort of depressed women. Arch Womens Ment Health 2013;16(6):465–73.
6. Goyal D, Gay C, Lee K. How much does low socioeconomic status increase the risk of prenatal and postpartum depressive symptoms in first-time mothers? Womens Health Issues 2010;20(2):96–104.
7. Le Strat Y, Dubertret C, Le Foll B. Prevalence and correlates of major depressive episode in pregnant and postpartum women in the United States. J Affect Dis-ord 2011;135(1):128–38.
8. Fortner R, Pekow P, Dole N, et al. Risk factors for prenatal depressive symptoms among hispanic women. Matern Child Health J 2011;15(8):1287–95.
9. Venkatesh K, Phipps M, Triche E, et al. The relationship between parental stress and postpartum depression among adolescent mothers enrolled in a random-ized controlled prevention trial. Matern Child Health J 2014;18(6):1532–9.
10. Schachman K, Lindsey L. A resilience perspective of postpartum depressive symptomatology in military wives. J Obstet Gynecol Neonatal Nurs 2013; 42(2):157–67.
11. Pinheiro R, Coelho F, Azevedo da Silva R, et al. Association of a serotonin trans-porter gene polymorphism (5-HTTLPR) and stressful life events with postpartum depressive symptoms: a population-based study. J Psychosom Obstet Gynae-col 2013;34(1):29–33.
12. Mrazek P, Haggerty R. Risk and protective factors for the onset of mental disorders. Washington, DC: National Academic Press; 1994.
13. Heneghan A, Silver E, Bauman L, et al. Depressive symptoms in inner-city mothers of young children: who is at risk? Pediatrics 1998;102(6):1394–400.

14. Cox J, Holden J, Sagovsky R. Detection of postnatal depression. Development of the 10-item Edinburgh postnatal depression scale. Br J Psychiatry 1987; 150(6):782–6.

15. Siegenthaler E, Munder T, Egger M. Effect of preventive interventions in mentally ill parents on the mental health of the offspring: systematic review and meta-analysis. J Am Acad Child Adolesc Psychiatry 2012;51(1):8–17.e18.

16. Gunlicks M, Weissman M. Change in child psychopathology with improvement in parental depression: a systematic review. J Am Acad Child Adolesc Psychiatry 2008;47(4):379–89.

17. Forman DR, O'hara MW, Stuart S, et al. Effective treatment for postpartum depression is not sufficient to improve the developing mother–child relationship. Dev Psychopathol 2007;19(2):585–602.

18. El Marroun H, White T, Verhulst F, et al. Maternal use of antidepressant or anxiolytic medication during pregnancy and childhood neurodevelopmental outcomes: a systematic review. Eur Child Adolesc Psychiatry 2014;23(10): 973–92.

19. Nulman I, Koren G, Rovet J, et al. Neurodevelopment of children prenatally exposed to selective reuptake inhibitor antidepressants: Toronto sibling study. J Clin Psychiatry 2015;76(7):e842–7.

20. Yonkers K, Wisner K, Stewart D, et al. The management of depression during pregnancy: a report from the American psychiatric association and the American college of obstetricians and gynecologists. Gen Hosp Psychiatry 2009; 31(5):403–13.

21. Drury S, Cuthbert B. Advancing pediatric psychiatry research linking neurobiological processes to novel treatment and diagnosis through the research domain criteria (RDoC) Project. Ther Innov Regul Sci 2015;49(5):643–6.

22. Poobalan A, Aucott L, Ross L, et al. Effects of treating postnatal depression on mother–infant interaction and child development. Br J Psychiatry 2007;191(5): 378–86.

23. Brett Z, Humphreys K, Fleming A, et al. Using cross species comparisons and a neurobiological framework to understand early social deprivation effects on behavioral development. Dev Psychopathol 2015;27:347–67.

24. Drury S, Scheeringa M, Schmidt K, et al. From biology to behavior to the Law: policy implications of the neurobiology of early adverse experiences. Whittier Journal of Child & Family Advocacy 2010;10(25).

25. Drury S, Gonzalez A, Sanchez M. When mothering goes awry: challenges and opportunities for utilizing evidence across rodent, primate and human studies to better define the biological consequences of negative early caregiving. Horm Behav 2015. [Epub ahead of print].

26. Stein A, Pearson R, Goodman S, et al. Effects of perinatal mental disorders on the fetus and child. Lancet 2014;384(9956):1800–19.

27. Howell B, Sanchez M. Understanding behavioral effects of early life stress using the reactive scope and allostatic load models. Dev Psychopathol 2011;23(4): 1001–16.

28. Raineki C, Lucion AB, Weinberg J. Neonatal handling: an overview of the positive and negative effects. Dev Psychobiol 2014;56(8):1613–25.

29. Rincon-Cortes M, Sullivan R. Early life trauma and attachment: immediate and enduring effects on neurobehavioral and stress axis development. Front Endocrinol (Lausanne) 2014;5:33.

30. Hofer M. Relationships as regulators: a psychobiologic perspective on bereavement. Psychosom Med 1984;46:183–97.

31. Kuhn CM, Schanberg SM, Field T, et al. Tactile-kinesthetic stimulation effects on sympathetic and adrenocortical function in preterm infants. J Pediatr 1991;119: 434–40.

32. Seyfried L, Marcus S. Postpartum mood disorders. Int Rev Psychiatry 2003; 15(3):231–42.

33. Josefsson A, Berg G, Nordin C, et al. Prevalence of depressive symptoms in late pregnancy and postpartum. Acta Obstet Gynecol Scand 2001;80(3):251–5.

34. Clay E, Seehusen D. A review of postpartum depression for the primary care physician. South Med J 2004;97(2):157–61 [quiz: 162].

35. Brockington I, Cernik K, Schofield E, et al. Puerperal psychosis: phenomena and diagnosis. Arch Gen Psychiatry 1981;38(7):829–33.

36. Benvenuti P, Cabras P, Servi P, et al. Puerperal psychoses: a clinical case study with follow-up. J Affect Disord 1992;26(1):25–30.

37. Kendell R, Chalmers J, Platz C. Epidemiology of puerperal psychoses. Br J Psychiatry 1987;150(5):662–73.

38. Patel V, DeSouza N, Rodrigues M. Postnatal depression and infant growth and development in low income countries: a cohort study from Goa, India. Arch Dis Child 2003;88(1):34–7.

39. Bauer A, Pawlby S, Plant D, et al. Perinatal depression and child development: exploring the economic consequences from a south London cohort. Psychol Med 2015;45(01):51–61.

40. Petrou S, Morrell C, Knapp M. An overview of health economic aspects of perinatal depression. identifying perinatal depression and anxiety: evidence-based practice in screening, psychosocial assessment, and management. West Sussex, UK: John Wiley and Sons; 2015. p. 228–39.

41. Brand S, Brennan P. Impact of antenatal and postpartum maternal mental illness: how are the children? Clin Obstet Gynecol 2009;52(3):441–55.

42. Conroy S, Pariante C, Marks M, et al. Maternal psychopathology and infant development at 18 months: the impact of maternal personality disorder and depression. J Am Acad Child Adolesc Psychiatry 2012;51(1):51–61.

43. Murray L, Arteche A, Fearon P, et al. Maternal postnatal depression and the development of depression in offspring up to 16 years of age. J Am Acad Child Adolesc Psychiatry 2011;50(5):460–70.

44. Verbeek T, Bockting C, van Pampus M, et al. Postpartum depression predicts offspring mental health problems in adolescence independently of parental life-time psychopathology. J Affect Disord 2012;136(3):948–54.

45. Naicker K, Wickham M, Colman I. Timing of first exposure to maternal depression and adolescent emotional disorder in a national Canadian cohort. PLoS One 2012;7(3):e33422.

46. Hernandez-Reif M, Field T, Diego M, et al. Greater arousal and less attentiveness to face/voice stimuli by neonates of depressed mothers on the brazelton neonatal behavioral assessment scale. Infant Behav Dev 2006;29(4):594–8.

47. Avan B, Richter L, Ramchandani P, et al. Maternal postnatal depression and children's growth and behaviour during the early years of life: exploring the interaction between physical and mental health. Arch Dis Child 2010;95(9):690–5.

48. Galéra C, Côté S, Bouvard M, et al. Early risk factors for hyperactivity-impulsivity and inattention trajectories from age 17 months to 8 years. Arch Gen Psychiatry 2011;68(12):1267–75.

49. Cornish A, McMahon C, Ungerer J, et al. Postnatal depression and infant cognitive and motor development in the second postnatal year: the impact of depression chronicity and infant gender. Infant Behav Dev 2005;28(4):407–17.

50. Feldman R, Granat A, Pariente C, et al. Maternal depression and anxiety across the postpartum year and infant social engagement, fear regulation, and stress reactivity. J Am Acad Child Adolesc Psychiatry 2009;48(9):919–27.
51. Murray L. The impact of postnatal depression on infant development. J Child Psychol Psychiatry 1992;33(3):543–61.
52. Brennan P, Pargas R, Walker E, et al. Maternal depression and infant cortisol: influences of timing, comorbidity and treatment. J Child Psychol Psychiatry 2008;49(10):1099–107.
53. Barry TJ, Murray L, Fearon R, et al. Maternal postnatal depression predicts altered offspring biological stress reactivity in adulthood. Psychoneuroendocrinology 2015;52:251–60.
54. Essex MJ, Klein MH, Cho E, et al. Maternal stress beginning in infancy may sensitize children to later stress exposure: effects on cortisol and behavior. Biol Psychiatry 2002;52(8):776–84.
55. Beck C. The effects of postpartum depression on maternal-infant interaction: a meta-analysis. Nurs Res 1995;44(5):298–305.
56. Rahman A, Iqbal Z, Bunn J, et al. Impact of maternal depression on infant nutritional status and illness: a cohort study. Arch Gen Psychiatry 2004;61(9): 946–52.
57. Deave T, Heron J, Evans J, et al. The impact of maternal depression in pregnancy on early child development. BJOG 2008;115(8):1043–51.
58. Byrne E, Carrillo-Roa T, Penninx B, et al. Applying polygenic risk scores to postpartum depression. Arch Womens Ment Health 2014;17(6):519–28.
59. Giallo R, Cooklin A, Wade C, et al. Maternal postnatal mental health and later emotional–behavioural development of children: the mediating role of parenting behaviour. Child Care Health Dev 2014;40(3):327–36.
60. Lovejoy C, Graczyk P, O'Hare E, et al. Maternal depression and parenting behavior: a meta-analytic review. Clin Psychol Rev 2000;20(5):561–92.
61. Olino T, McMakin D, Nicely T, et al. Maternal depression, parenting, and youth depressive symptoms: mediation and moderation in a short-term longitudinal study. J Clin Child Adolesc Psychol 2015;1–12 [Epub ahead of print].
62. Tomlinson M, Cooper P, Murray L. The Mother–Infant relationship and infant attachment in a South African Peri-Urban settlement. Child Dev 2005;76(5): 1044–54.
63. Van Ijzendoorn M, Schuengel C, Bakermans-Kranenburg M. Disorganized attachment in early childhood: meta-analysis of precursors, concomitants, and sequelae. Dev Psychopathol 1999;11(02):225–50.
64. McLearn K, Minkovitz C, Strobino D, et al. Maternal depressive symptoms at 2 to 4 months post partum and early parenting practices. Arch Pediatr Adolesc Med 2006;160(3):279–84.
65. Cadzow S, Armstrong K, Fraser J. Stressed parents with infants: reassessing physical abuse risk factors. Child Abuse Negl 1999;23(9):845–53.
66. Egami E, Ford D, Greenfield S, et al. Psychiatric profile and sociodemographic characteristics of adults who report physically abusing or neglecting children. Am J Psychiatry 1996;153(7):921–8.
67. Éthier L, Lacharité C, Couture G. Childhood adversity, parental stress, and depression of negligent mothers. Child Abuse Negl 1995;19(5):619–32.
68. Tyler S, Allison K, Winsler A. Child neglect: developmental consequences, intervention, and policy implications. Presented at the Child and Youth Care Forum. 2006.

69. Lyons-Ruth K, Lyubchik A, Wolfe R, et al. Parental depression and child attachment: hostile and helpless profiles of parent and child behavior among families at risk. 2002.

70. Bradley R, Whiteside-Mansell L, Brisby J, et al. Parents' socioemotional investment in children. J Marriage Fam 1997;59(1):77–90.

71. Bird C. Gender differences in the social and economic burdens of parenting and psychological distress. J Marriage Fam 1997;59(4):809–23.

72. Turney K. Labored love: examining the link between maternal depression and parenting behaviors. Soc Sci Res 2011;40(1):399–415.

73. Bodovski K, Youn M. Love, discipline and elementary school achievement: the role of family emotional climate. Soc Sci Res 2010;39(4):585–95.

74. Minkovitz C, Strobino D, Scharfstein D, et al. Maternal depressive symptoms and children's receipt of health care in the first 3 years of life. Pediatrics 2005; 115(2):306–14.

75. Kiernan K, Huerta M. Economic deprivation, maternal depression, parenting and children's cognitive and emotional development in early childhood1. Br J Sociol 2008;59(4):783–806.

76. Myers E, Aubuchon-Endsley N, Bastian L, et al. Efficacy and safety of screening for postpartum depression. Rockville, MD: Agency for Health Care Research and Quality; 2013.

77. Sejourne N, Alba J, Onorrus M, et al. Intergenerational transmission of postpartum depression. J Reprod Infant Psychol 2011;29(2):115–24.

78. Goodman S, Gotlib I. Risk for psychopathology in the children of depressed mothers: a developmental model for understanding mechanisms of transmission. Psychol Rev 1999;106(3):458–90.

79. Buist A. Childhood abuse, parenting and postpartum depression. Aust N Z J Psychiatry 1998;32(4):479–87.

80. Buist A, Janson H. Childhood sexual abuse, parenting and postpartum depression—a 3-year follow-up study. Child Abuse Negl 2001;25(7):909–21.

81. Chaudron L, Szilagyi P, Kitzman H, et al. Detection of postpartum depressive symptoms by screening at well-child visits. Pediatrics 2004;113(3):551–8.

82. World Health Organization. WHO recommendations on postnatal care of the mother and newborn. Geneva, Switzerland: World Health Organization; 2014.

83. Tandon S, Cluxton-Keller F, Leis J, et al. A comparison of three screening tools to identify perinatal depression among low-income African American women. J Affect Disord 2012;136(1–2):155–62.

84. Gaynes B, Gavin N, Meltzer-Brody S, et al. Perinatal depression: prevalence, screening accuracy, and screening outcomes. Evid Rep Technol Assess (Summ) 2005;(119):1–8.

85. Whitton A, Warner R, Appleby L. The pathway to care in post-natal depression: women's attitudes to post-natal depression and its treatment. Br J Gen Pract 1996;46(408):427–8.

86. Goodman J, Tyer-Viola L. Detection, treatment, and referral of perinatal depression and anxiety by obstetrical providers. J Womens Health 2010; 19(3):477–90.

87. LaRocco-Cockburn A, Melville J, Bell M, et al. Depression screening attitudes and practices among obstetrician–gynecologists. Obstet Gynecol 2003; 101(5 Pt 1):892–8.

88. Liberto T. Screening for depression and help-seeking in postpartum women during well-baby pediatric visits: an integrated review. J Pediatr Health Care 2012; 26(2):109–17.

89. Dennis C. Preventing postpartum depression part II: a critical review of nonbiological interventions. Can J Psychiatry 2004;49:526–38.

90. Dennis C, Hodnett E, Kenton L, et al. Effect of peer support on prevention of postnatal depression among high risk women: multisite randomised controlled trial. BMJ 2009;338:a3064.

91. Sockol L, Epperson C, Barber J. Preventing postpartum depression: a meta-analytic review. Clin Psychol Rev 2013;33(8):1205–17.

92. Morrell C, Spiby H, Stewart P, et al. Costs and effectiveness of community postnatal support workers: randomised controlled trial. BMJ 2000;321(7261):593–8.

93. Werner E, Miller M, Osborne L, et al. Preventing postpartum depression: review and recommendations. Arch Womens Ment Health 2015;18(1):41–60.

94. Barlow J, Stewart-Brown S. Costs and effectiveness of community postnatal support workers: researchers must now focus on effectiveness with specific groups of women. BMJ 2001;322(7281):301.

95. MacArthur C, Winter H, Bick D, et al. Effects of redesigned community postnatal care on womens' health 4 months after birth: a cluster randomised controlled trial. Lancet 2002;359(9304):378–85.

96. Dukhovny D, Dennis C, Hodnett E, et al. Prospective economic evaluation of a peer support intervention for prevention of postpartum depression among high-risk women in Ontario, Canada. Am J Perinatol 2013;30(8):631–42.

97. Shaw E, Levitt C, Wong S, et al, The McMaster University Postpartum Research Group. Systematic review of the literature on postpartum care: effectiveness of postpartum support to improve maternal parenting, mental health, quality of life, and physical health. Birth 2006;33(3):210–20.

98. Brugha T, Morrell C, Slade P, et al. Universal prevention of depression in women postnatally: cluster randomized trial evidence in primary care. Psychol Med 2011;41(4):739–48.

99. Sockol L. A systematic review of the efficacy of cognitive behavioral therapy for treating and preventing perinatal depression. J Affect Disord 2015;177:7–21.

100. Dennis C. Psychosocial and psychological interventions for prevention of postnatal depression: systematic review. BMJ 2005;331(7507):15.

101. Ertel K, Rich-Edwards J, Koenen K. Maternal depression in the United States: nationally representative rates and risks. J Womens Health (Larchmt) 2011; 20(11):1609–17.

102. Dudas R, Csatordai S, Devosa I, et al. Obstetric and psychosocial risk factors for depressive symptoms during pregnancy. Psychiatry Res 2012;200(2):323–8.

103. Jackson C, Drury S, Jacobs M, et al. Maternal cumulative life course stress and child psychopathology, in press.

104. Choi K, Sikkema K. Childhood maltreatment and perinatal mood and anxiety disorders a systematic review. Trauma Violence Abuse 2015. [Epub ahead of print].

105. Hillis S, Anda R, Dube S, et al. The association between adverse childhood experiences and adolescent pregnancy, long-term psychosocial consequences, and fetal death. Pediatrics 2004;113(2):320–7.

106. Gavin A, Thompson E, Rue T, et al. Maternal early life risk factors for offspring birth weight: findings from the add health study. Prev Sci 2012;13(2):162–72.

107. Plant D, Barker ED, Waters C, et al. Intergenerational transmission of maltreatment and psychopathology: the role of antenatal depression. Psychol Med 2013;43(3):519–28.

108. Roberts A, Chen Y, Slopen N, et al. Maternal experience of abuse in childhood and depressive symptoms in adolescent and adult offspring: a 21 year long study. Depress Anxiety 2015;32(10):709–19.

109. Tahirkheli N, Cherry A, Tackett A, et al. Postpartum depression on the neonatal intensive care unit: current perspectives. Int J Womens Health 2014;6:975.
110. Vasa R, Eldeirawi K, Kuriakose V, et al. Postpartum depression in mothers of infants in neonatal intensive care unit: risk factors and management strategies. Am J Perinatol 2014;31(5):425–34
111. Silverstein M, Feinberg E, Cabral H, et al. Problem-solving education to prevent depression among low-income mothers of preterm infants: a randomized controlled pilot trial. Arch Womens Ment Health 2011;14(4):317–24.
112. Meyer E, Coll C, Lester B, et al. Family-based intervention improves maternal psychological well-being and feeding interaction of preterm infants. Pediatrics 1994;93(2):241–6.
113. Hagan R, Evans S, Pope S. Preventing postnatal depression in mothers of very preterm infants: a randomised controlled trial. BJOG 2004;111(7):641–7.
114. Brecht C, Shaw R, St John N, et al. Effectiveness of therapeutic and behavioral interventions for parents of low-birth-weight premature infants: a review. Infant Ment Health J 2012;33(6):651–65.
115. Brisch K, Bechinger D, Betzler S, et al. Early preventive attachment-oriented psychotherapeutic intervention program with parents of a very low birthweight premature infant: results of attachment and neurological development. Attach Hum Dev 2003;5(2):120–35.
116. Newnham C, Milgrom J, Skouteris H. Effectiveness of a modified mother–infant transaction program on outcomes for preterm infants from 3 to 24 months of age. Infant Behav Dev 2009;32(1):17–26.
117. Rauh V, Achenbach T, Nurcombe B, et al. Minimizing adverse effects of low birthweight: four-year results of an early intervention program. Child Dev 1988;59(3):544–53.
118. Rahkonen P, Heinonen K, Pesonen A, et al. Mother-child interaction is associated with neurocognitive outcome in extremely low gestational age children. Scand J Psychol 2014;55(4):311–8.
119. Bilgin A, Wolke D. Maternal sensitivity in parenting preterm children: a meta-analysis. Pediatrics 2015;136(1):e177–93.
120. Werner E, Gustafsson H, Lee S, et al. PREPP: postpartum depression prevention through the mother–infant dyad. Arch Womens Ment Health 2015;1–14 [Epub ahead of print].
121. Danaher B, Milgrom J, Seeley J, et al. Web-based intervention for postpartum depression: formative research and design of the MomMoodBooster program. JMIR Res Protoc 2012;1(2):e18.
122. Haga S, Drozd F, Brendryen H, et al. Mamma mia: a feasibility study of a Web-based intervention to reduce the risk of postpartum depression and enhance subjective well-being. JMIR Res Protoc 2013;2(2):e29.
123. Danaher B, Milgrom J, Seeley J, et al. MomMoodBooster web-based intervention for postpartum depression: feasibility trial results. J Med Internet Res 2013;15(11):e242.
124. Osma J, Plaza I, Crespo E, et al. Proposal of use of smartphones to evaluate and diagnose depression and anxiety symptoms during pregnancy and after birth. Presented at the Biomedical and Health Informatics (BHI), 2014 IEEE-EMBS International Conference on 2014. Valencia (Spain), June 1–4, 2014.
125. Barrera A, Wickham R, Muñoz R. Online prevention of postpartum depression for Spanish-and English-speaking pregnant women: a pilot randomized controlled trial. Internet Interv 2015;2(3):257–65.

126. Shaw D, Connell A, Dishion T, et al. Improvements in maternal depression as a mediator of intervention effects on early childhood problem behavior. Dev Psychopathol 2009;21(2):417–39.

127. O'Mahen H, Himle J, Fedock G, et al. A pilot randomized controlled trial of cognitive behavioral therapy for perinatal depression adapted for women with low incomes. Depress Anxiety 2013;30(7):679–87.

128. Urizar G, Muñoz R. Impact of a prenatal cognitive-behavioral stress management intervention on salivary cortisol levels in low-income mothers and their infants. Psychoneuroendocrinology 2011;36(10):1480–94.

129. Mendelson T, Leis J, Perry D, et al. Impact of a preventive intervention for perinatal depression on mood regulation, social support, and coping. Arch Womens Ment Health 2013;16(3):211–8.

130. O'Mahen H, Richards D, Woodford J, et al. Netmums: a phase II randomized controlled trial of a guided internet behavioural activation treatment for postpartum depression. Psychol Med 2014;44(08):1675–89.

131. Tandon S, Perry D, Mendelson T, et al. Preventing perinatal depression in low-income home visiting clients: a randomized controlled trial. J Consult Clin Psychol 2011;79(5):707.

132. Letourneau N, Stewart M, Dennis C, et al. Effect of home-based peer support on maternal–infant interactions among women with postpartum depression: a randomized, controlled trial. Int J Ment Health Nurs 2011;20(5):345–57.

133. Morrell C, Warner R, Slade P, et al. Psychological interventions for postnatal depression: cluster randomised trial and economic evaluation. The PoNDER trial. Health Technol Assess 2009;13(30):iii–iv, xi–xiii, 1–153.

134. Gilkerson L, Gray L, Mork N. Fussy babies, worried families and a new service network. Zero to Three 2005;25:34–41. Available at: aia.berkeley.edu/strengthening_connections/handouts/3a/Zero to three article.pdf. Accessed December 19, 2015.

135. Hiscock H, Bayer J, Hampton A, et al. Long-term mother and child mental health effects of a population-based infant sleep intervention: cluster-randomized, controlled trial. Pediatrics 2008;122(3):e621–7.

136. Wake M, Morton-Allen E, Poulakis Z, et al. Prevalence, stability, and outcomes of cry-fuss and sleep problems in the first 2 years of life: prospective community-based study. Pediatrics 2006;117(3):836–42.

137. Buist A. Childhood abuse, postpartum depression and parenting difficulties: a literature review of associations. Aust N Z J Psychiatry 1998;32(3):370–8.

138. Hiscock H, Cook F, Bayer J, et al. Preventing early infant sleep and crying problems and postnatal depression: a randomized trial. Pediatrics 2014;133(2):e346–54.

139. Mindell J, Telofski L, Wiegand B, et al. A nightly bedtime routine: impact on sleep in young children and maternal mood. Sleep 2009;32(5):599–606.

140. Yim I, Glynn L, Schetter C, et al. Risk of postpartum depressive symptoms with elevated corticotropin-releasing hormone in human pregnancy. Arch Gen Psychiatry 2009;66(2):162–9.

141. Yim I, Tanner Stapleton L, Guardino C, et al. Biological and psychosocial predictors of postpartum depression: systematic review and call for integration. Annu Rev Clin Psychol 2015;11:99–137.

142. Cuijpers P, Brannmark J, Straten A. Psychological treatment of postpartum depression: a meta-analysis. J Clin Psychol 2008;64(1):103–18.

143. Dimidjian S, Goodman S. Nonpharmacologic intervention and prevention strategies for depression during pregnancy and the postpartum. Clin Obstet Gynecol 2009;52(3):498–515.

144. Murray L, Cooper P, Wilson A, et al. Controlled trial of the short-and long-term effect of psychological treatment of post-partum depression 2. Impact on the mother—child relationship and child outcome. Br J Psychiatry 2003;182(5): 420–7.

145. Toth S, Rogosch F, Manly J, et al. The efficacy of toddler-parent psychotherapy to reorganize attachment in the young offspring of mothers with major depressive disorder: a randomized preventive trial. J Consult Clin Psychol 2006; 74(6):1006.

146. Cuijpers P, Weitz E, Karyotaki E, et al. The effects of psychological treatment of maternal depression on children and parental functioning: a meta-analysis. Eur Child Adolesc Psychiatry 2015;24(2):237–45.

147. Toth S, Rogosch F, Oshri A, et al. The efficacy of interpersonal psychotherapy for depression among economically disadvantaged mothers. Dev Psychopathol 2013;25(4 Pt 1):1065–78.

148. Mulcahy R, Reay R, Wilkinson R, et al. A randomised control trial for the effectiveness of group interpersonal psychotherapy for postnatal depression. Arch Womens Ment Health 2010;13(2):125–39.

149. Spinelli MG, Endicott J. Controlled clinical trial of interpersonal psychotherapy versus parenting education program for depressed pregnant women. Am J Psychiatry 2003;160(3):555–62.

150. Cicchetti D, Toth S, Handley E. Genetic moderation of interpersonal psychotherapy efficacy for low-income mothers with major depressive disorder: implications for differential susceptibility. Dev Psychopathol 2015;27(1):19–35.

151. Cooper P, Murray L, Wilson A, et al. Controlled trial of the short-and long-term effect of psychological treatment of post-partum depression. Br J Psychiatry 2003;182(5):412–9.

152. Verduyn C, Barrowclough C, Roberts J, et al. Maternal depression and child behaviour problems Randomised placebo-controlled trial of a cognitive–behavioural group intervention. Br J Psychiatry 2003;183(4):342–8.

153. van den Heuvel M, Johannos M, Henrichs J, et al. Maternal mindfulness during pregnancy and infant socio-emotional development and temperament: the mediating role of maternal anxiety. Early Hum Dev 2015;91(2): 103–8.

154. Tsivos Z, Calam R, Sanders M, et al. Interventions for postnatal depression assessing the mother–infant relationship and child developmental outcomes: a systematic review. Int J Womens Health 2015;7:429.

155. Cicchetti D, Rogosch F, Toth S. The efficacy of toddler-parent psychotherapy for fostering cognitive development in offspring of depressed mothers. J Abnorm Child Psychol 2000;28(2):135–48.

156. Lavi I, Gard A, Hagan M, et al. Child-parent psychotherapy examined in a perinatal sample: depression, posttraumatic stress symptoms and child-rearing attitudes. J Soc Clin Psychol 2015;34(1):64–82.

157. Tsivos Z, Calam R, Sanders M, et al. A pilot randomised controlled trial to evaluate the feasibility and acceptability of the Baby Triple P positive parenting programme in mothers with postnatal depression. Clin Child Psychol Psychiatry 2015;20(4):532–54.

158. Onozawa K, Glover V, Adams D, et al. Infant massage improves mother–infant interaction for mothers with postnatal depression. J Affect Disord 2001;63(1): 201–7.

159. Glover V, Onozawa K, Hodgkinson A. Benefits of infant massage for mothers with postnatal depression. Semin Neonatol 2002;7(6):495–500.

160. O'Higgins M, St James Roberts I, Glover V. Postnatal depression and mother and infant outcomes after infant massage. J Affect Disord 2008;109(1–2): 189–92.
161. Morhenn V, Beavin L, Zak P. Massage increases oxytocin and reduces adrenocorticotropin hormone in humans. Altern Ther Health Med 2012;18(6): 11–8.
162. Moyer C, Seefeldt L, Mann E, et al. Does massage therapy reduce cortisol? A comprehensive quantitative review. J Bodyw Mov Ther 2011;15(1):3–14.

Prevention of Depression in Childhood and Adolescence

Tamar Mendelson, PhD[a],*, S. Darius Tandon, PhD[b]

KEYWORDS

- Prevention • Children • Adolescents • Depressive symptoms • Depressive disorder
- Intervention

KEY POINTS

- Depression prevention with children and adolescents is a vital public health goal with potential to improve population health and reduce health care costs.
- Depression prevention programs can be implemented using universal, selective, and indicated approaches in a range of settings (eg, schools, family contexts, primary care).
- Universal and targeted depression prevention programs produce small but significant effects that compare favorably with other types of youth-focused prevention, including substance abuse and human immunodeficiency virus prevention.
- Future studies should include rigorous design features, including attention control groups, long-term follow-up assessments, and tests of moderation and mediation.
- The next critical phase in research on depression prevention for young people will focus on effectiveness trials assessing dissemination and implementation.

INTRODUCTION

Depression is the most common psychiatric disorder and one of the leading causes of morbidity and mortality in the United States. Nationally representative epidemiologic studies indicate that the lifetime prevalence of depression among adolescents aged 15 to 18 years is between 11% and 14%, with an estimated 20% of adolescents experiencing major depression disorder (MDD) by the time they turn 18 years.[1,2] It is also estimated that approximately half of first episodes of depression occur during adolescence.[3] In addition, approximately one-quarter of adolescents endorse subthreshold depressive symptoms that cause impairment in daily functioning.[4] MDD in

Disclosure: The authors have nothing to disclose.
[a] Department of Mental Health, Johns Hopkins Bloomberg School of Public Health, 624 North Broadway, Room 853, Baltimore, MD 21205, USA; [b] Department of Medical Social Sciences, Institute for Public Health and Medicine, Northwestern University Feinberg School of Medicine, Rubloff Building, 6th Floor, 750 Lake Shore Drive, Chicago, IL 60611, USA
* Corresponding author.
E-mail address: Tmendel1@jhu.edu

Child Adolesc Psychiatric Clin N Am 25 (2016) 201–218
http://dx.doi.org/10.1016/j.chc.2015.11.005
1056-4993/16/$ – see front matter © 2016 Elsevier Inc. All rights reserved.

childpsych.theclinics.com

adolescents is associated with difficulties in relationships, increased risk for substance use, increased rates of suicide, and impaired school performance.[5] Both MDD and subthreshold depressive symptoms during adolescence are associated with greater prospective risk of MDD.[6,7]

Rationale for Prevention

The term prevention refers to interventions administered before the onset of a clinically diagnosable disorder, in contrast with treatment, which refers to services designed to improve or cure an existing disorder.[8] There are effective psychosocial and pharmacologic treatments for depression,[9] so why is the prevention of depression an important public health goal?

Prevention is critical in part because of limitations associated with treatment availability, access to care, and the impact of depression on overall health. There is an insufficient number of providers (particularly in low-resource global settings) to treat all individuals who have depression.[10] Several other barriers also impede service use, including attitudinal factors (eg, stigma) and structural barriers (eg, distance from appropriate facilities, unavailability of linguistically and culturally appropriate services, financial constraints).[11] Moreover, not everyone with depression responds to treatment; research indicates that up to one-third of patients do not improve following treatment of depression.[12] It has been estimated that, even under optimal conditions, depression treatment is not able to avert more than 50% of the burden of disability-adjusted life years lost[13] or 23% of the burden of years lived with disability.[14]

Prevention of depression offers opportunities for improving long-term emotional and physical outcomes and overall functioning. First episodes of depression generally occur during adolescence or young adulthood.[3] Prevention and early intervention can boost a young person's chance of healthy social and emotional development during these critical developmental phases. Depression co-occurs with other physical and mental health problems, including chronic physical diseases, substance use, and anxiety disorders.[15–17] Preventing depression may thus delay or prevent the subsequent onset of a second comorbid disorder, improving a person's functioning across multiple domains. Depression is also a chronic disorder with a recurrence rate of approximately 50% after a single episode, 70% after 2 episodes, and 90% after 3 episodes.[18,19] Preventing or delaying an initial depressive episode may thus significantly reduce lifetime mental health care needs.[20] Prevention may offer significant cost savings[21] that result from the impact of mental disorders on affected individuals, as well as their families and other members of society.[20,22,23] Savings may include health care costs, reduced productivity and missed days at work, costs to the criminal justice and juvenile justice systems, and costs associated with lost educational opportunities and need for special education. In addition, reducing potential suffering caused by depression at a population level is consistent with the mission of public health and with humanitarian values (**Box 1**).[24,25]

A Framework for Prevention

Prevention scientists have argued for the importance of an integrated interdisciplinary framework for prevention of mental disorders that includes epidemiology, life-course development, and experimental trial methodology.[26] Development of effective interventions to prevent depression, for instance, depends on epidemiologic methods to identify risk and protective factors for depression and their distribution across time, place, and individuals. Life-course development theory shapes research on the timing and trajectories of risk and protective factors and disorders, informing decisions about which factors are most malleable and which developmental time periods may be

> **Box 1**
> **Rationale for depression prevention**
>
> - Clinicians do not have sufficient resources to treat all individuals with depression
> - Depression treatment is not effective for everyone
> - Depression prevention can increase opportunities for healthy development across multiple domains
> - Depression prevention reduces lifetime mental health care needs and likely saves money
> - Preventing suffering is ethical and humane

critical, sensitive, or optimal for prevention or early intervention. Well-designed randomized controlled trials are the gold standard for assessing efficacy of preventive interventions,[27] and findings from these trials can help refine developmental theories regarding pathways to disorder.[28]

There is a large empirical literature on risk and protective factors for depression to inform the development of depression prevention programs and to guide decisions about the timing of intervention delivery and the selection of target child and adolescent populations. As described by Gladstone and colleagues,[29] some risk factors are specific to depression, whereas others are nonspecific, meaning that they are associated with greater likelihood of developing a range of mental health problems, including depression. Specific risk factors for child and adolescent depression include having a parent with depression (the most robust risk factor) as well as low self-esteem, negative body image, maladaptive cognitive style, low social support, poor coping skills, and female gender.[30,31] Nonspecific risk factors include poverty, violence exposure, child maltreatment, and family instability.[30,31] Factors known to buffer against development of depression (protective factors) include effective coping and self-regulation skills and supportive relationships.[30] Interventions to prevent depression typically target one or more of these risk and protective factors. Some risk factors, such as negative cognitive style, are known to be malleable; others, such as having a parent with depression or being female, can be addressed by selecting youth with these characteristics to target for prevention efforts. Given that risk for depressive symptoms and disorders increases steeply during puberty,[1,3] most depression prevention programs target preadolescent or early adolescent youth.

Types of Prevention

The Institute of Medicine defined 3 categories of preventive intervention.[32] Universal preventive interventions target an entire population group (eg, a school-wide depression prevention program). Selective preventive interventions target subgroups at risk for development of the disorder, using empirically identified biological, psychological, or social indicators of risk to select appropriate subgroups (eg, a depression prevention program for children of depressed parents). Indicated preventive interventions target individuals at highest risk for developing the disorder based on subclinical symptoms or signs that do not yet meet full diagnostic criteria (eg, a depression prevention program for adolescents with subthreshold depression symptoms).[8] Recognizing that universal interventions may reduce risk factors and prevent adverse outcomes in some, but not all, individuals, a tiered approach in which children and adolescents who do not respond well to a universal intervention receive selective or indicated interventions is an alternative to focusing on just 1 of the Institute of Medicine categories.[33]

OVERVIEW OF PREVENTION SETTINGS AND PROGRAMS

Interventions to prevent depression in children and adolescents are delivered in settings that are central to young people's lives and development, including schools and family-oriented contexts. This article provides an overview of the types of programs that have been implemented and studied. This overview is not a systematic review; it is intended to offer a broad-based summary of the state of the field and to provide examples of the contents and outcomes of a few specific programs. Because most depression prevention programs for young people have been offered in schools, this article provides a more detailed discussion of this area, highlighting examples of school-based interventions that have been evaluated in randomized studies.

School-based Approaches

Most depression prevention programs for children and adolescents are implemented in school settings. Schools are a promising context for preventing depression, because most young people spend a large portion of their time in schools, and schools have potential for significant influences on child development.[34–36] A variety of school-based approaches have been implemented, including universal programs delivered to all students in a grade or school and targeted programs delivered either to students who have risk factors for depression (selective approaches) or those with subthreshold symptoms of depression (indicated approaches). There is also variability in how programs are implemented, with some delivered by trained mental health care professionals and others by school personnel without specialized mental health training.

Seven school-based interventions to prevent depression are discussed here; 3 evaluated as universal prevention approaches, 2 as selective, and 2 as indicated. These programs were selected because each was evaluated using a randomized design, and they provide a sense of the types of depression prevention programs commonly implemented. Some of these programs were found to be effective in randomized controlled studies, and others were not; these examples illustrate the heterogeneity in study designs and outcomes and the complexity of evaluating a prevention program's efficacy. **Table 1** provides a summary of key characteristics of each intervention.

Universal programs

Many depression prevention programs have been implemented universally. This article describes 3 that were evaluated in well-designed studies.

Resourceful adolescent program The Resourceful Adolescent Program (RAP)[37] was developed at Queensland University of Technology in Australia as a universal prevention program. The program is intended to reduce known risk factors for depression and promote protective factors. RAP-A (adolescent) is an 11-session school-based program delivered during the school day by psychologists or, in 1 study,[38] by teachers. RAP-F (family) is a modified version of the program in which students receive RAP-A with the addition of 3 family-focused sessions delivered by a psychologist.

Shochet and colleagues[39] designed a 3-armed randomized controlled trial comparing RAP-A versus RAP-F versus a no-intervention comparison group for reduction of adolescent depressive symptoms in a sample of 260 ninth-grade students. Participants in RAP-A and RAP-F reported significantly lower levels of depressive symptoms and hopelessness compared with participants in the control group. Addition of a family component (RAP-F) did not produce significantly better outcomes compared with RAP-A. Difficulty recruiting parents to participate highlighted feasibility issues with the parent component and also limited ability to evaluate the efficacy of RAP-F. The study supported the feasibility and acceptability of implementing RAP in school settings and provided encouraging data on the potential of the intervention to benefit both adolescents with initial depressive symptoms and those who seemed healthy at baseline.

Merry and colleagues[38] conducted a randomized controlled trial testing the efficacy of RAP-Kiwi, which was adapted from RAP for use with Maori and Pakeha adolescents, in 2 schools in New Zealand (n = 392 students). A strength of this study was the use of an active placebo control, a program matched on key characteristics such as length of the intervention but with no cognitive components for preventing depression. Both programs were teacher administered. Intervention participants improved relative to control participants on 2 measures of depressive symptoms at posttest and on 1 measure of depressive symptoms at the 18-month follow-up point. Findings suggested a small but significant intervention effect. More recent work found that the RAP intervention was feasible and acceptable to participants and school personnel in the United Kingdom,[40] suggesting potential for using the intervention in diverse contexts.

beyondblue The beyondblue initiative to prevent depression in adolescents uses a multicomponent school-based universal approach.[41] The intervention includes a 10-session curriculum delivered by teachers that provides instruction in problem solving, adaptive cognitive styles, social skills, and coping skills. Other components include a focus on building supportive environments to improve social interactions within the school community; building pathways for care and education by increasing student access to resources for mental health and other aspects of functioning; and creating community forums that provide information on mental health to students, families, and school personnel.

The intervention was tested in a randomized controlled trial that enrolled 5633 students in grade 8 across 50 secondary schools in Australia. Schools matched by socioeconomic status were randomized either to the intervention or a no-intervention comparison condition. Adolescents were exposed to the intervention over a 3-year period, and assessments were conducted annually over a 5-year period to evaluate intervention effects on protective factors (eg, optimistic thinking, problem solving), depressive symptoms, and school climate. No significant differences were found between the intervention and control schools on any of the targeted outcomes either following intervention implementation or over the additional 5 years of follow-up, except that teachers (but not students) reported improvements in school climate.[41,42] Challenges included implementation issues, such as training teachers to deliver the program with fidelity and promoting student engagement. It took an average of 2 years for schools to adequately integrate the school-level intervention components, highlighting the complexities of implementing and testing a whole-school approach.

Problem Solving for Life The 8-session Problem Solving for Life (PSFL) intervention uses cognitive restructuring and problem-solving approaches.[43,44] The program was evaluated in a randomized controlled trial implemented with 1500 grade 8 students across 16 schools in Queensland, Australia.[45] Schools were randomly allocated to the PSFL intervention or a no-intervention control group. Postintervention findings indicated that, compared with students in the comparison group, intervention students had decreased depressive symptom scores and improved problem-solving skills. This pattern was found both in students who had increased baseline depressive symptoms (high-risk group) and in those who did not (low-risk group).[45] There were no significant differences between the intervention and control groups at 12-month or at

Table 1
Sample school-based depression prevention programs

Program	Prevention Approach	Content/Core Components	Goal	Sample Selection	Ages (y)	Program Facilitators	Number and Length of Sessions
RAP	Universal	CBT (sessions 1–7) and IPT (sessions 8–10)	Enhance resilience via improved coping skills	All students	12–15	Psychologists (or teachers)	11 weekly sessions of 40–50 min
beyondblue	Universal	Curriculum Intervention; Building Supportive Environments; Building Pathways for Care and Education; community forums	Improve youth protective factors (social and coping skills) and reduce risk factors; improve school climate	All students	Year 8 students	Teachers	10 sessions of 40–45 min during 1 school term (for Curriculum Intervention)
PSFL	Universal	Cognitive restructuring and problem-solving skills training	Improve adolescents' ability to modify harmful thoughts and to use positive problem-solving skills	All students	Grade 8 students (12–14)	Teachers	8 sessions of 45–50 min delivered weekly
PRP	Selective	Cognitive behavioral skills to address links between thoughts and emotions and improve cognition and problem solving/coping	Reduce depressive symptoms by improving cognition and coping	Low-income and racial/ethnic minority students	10–14	Masters-level student and undergraduate psychology major	12 weekly sessions of 90 min

AOP	Selective	Optimistic thinking skills and social life skills	Reduce depression and anxiety symptoms by enhancing cognitive and social protective factors	Low-income students	11–13; grade 7	Teachers	20 weekly sessions of 60 min
The Feelings Club	Indicated	Cognitive behavioral skills, particularly cognitive restructuring, adapted from a treatment program for child anxiety	Reduce depressive and anxiety symptoms by improving cognitions and coping	Students screening positive for internalizing symptoms	Grades 3–6	Psychologists and psychology graduate students	12 weekly sessions of 90 min
PGC	Indicated	Based on strain, social learning, social control, and social support theories/perspectives; incorporates 2 core components: social support and life-skills training	Reduce depressive symptoms and suicide risk by enhancing social support and skills	Students screening positive for suicide risk	Grades 9–12	School teachers, counselors, or nurses	20 weekly sessions of 60 min

Abbreviations: AOP, Aussie Optimism Program; CBT, cognitive behavior therapy; IPT, interpersonal therapy; PGC, Personal Growth Class; PRP, Penn Resiliency Program; PSFL, Problem Solving for Life; RAP, Resourceful Adolescent Program.

2-year, 3-year, and 4-year follow-ups, with the exception of greater improvements in problem solving among high-risk intervention versus high-risk control participants, suggesting that intervention gains did not persist over time.[45,46]

Selective programs
Selective school-based programs target students with known risk factors for mental disorders in general, or depression in particular. Two interventions implemented with students at risk for mental health issues caused by economic disadvantage and/or minority race and ethnicity are discussed here.

Penn Resiliency Program The Penn Resiliency Program (PRP) (Gilham JE, Reivich KJ, Jaycox LH. The Penn Resiliency Program; unpublished work, 2008) is one of the most well-studied depression prevention programs to date, having been implemented and tested numerous times and replicated with different racial and ethnic groups. Unlike many other such programs, PRP has been implemented using both universal and targeted approaches.[47] PRP is a group cognitive behavioral prevention program for adolescents aged 10 to 14 years. The program is generally delivered in school settings but has also been implemented in other contexts, such as primary care and juvenile detention.[47]

Cardemil and colleagues[48,49] implemented PRP with low-income racial and ethnic minority children. Although the intervention was administered universally in the study schools and children were not screened individually for symptoms or risk factors, this work can be conceptualized as selective prevention given that low-income and ethnic minority status have been associated with risk for depressive symptoms[50–52] and other mental health problems.[29] Latino and African American students (n = 168) in 2 schools serving low-income communities were randomly assigned to a version of PRP tailored for low-income minority youth or to a no-intervention control group. Latino students in the intervention showed improvements in depressive symptoms relative to their counterparts in the control condition through the 6-month[48] and 2-year follow-up assessments.[49] Group differences were stronger at the 6-month follow-up, with additional improvements in negative cognitions and self-esteem. However, the African American students in the intervention did not show greater improvements relative to African American control students at any assessment point; both groups of African American students improved over time, a finding that merits additional study.[49]

Aussie Optimism Program The Aussie Optimism Program (AOP) is a school-based intervention to prevent depression and anxiety symptoms in adolescence, and is delivered by teachers as part of the school health curriculum. The program is hypothesized to reduce internalizing symptoms by addressing social and cognitive risk and protective factors associated with depression and anxiety. Specifically, the program includes 2 core components, one focused on teaching social life skills to improve interpersonal functioning,[53] and the other focused on optimistic thinking skills to improve attributional style, self-perceptions, problem solving, and coping.[54] AOP has been implemented in a selective manner by offering the program at schools serving low-income communities, in which students are exposed to poverty-related stressors, including financial challenges, single-parent families, and housing instability.

Roberts and colleagues[55] conducted a randomized controlled trial with 496 grade 7 students at 12 government schools serving disadvantaged areas in Perth, Western Australia. Schools were randomly assigned either to AOP or to standard health education classes. Students in the intervention group showed significant improvement in parent-rated internalizing symptoms, but not self-reported measures, at posttest. No differences between the study groups were evident at 6-month or 18-month follow-up assessments. The intervention was acceptable to students and school personnel, and intervention fidelity was high, suggesting that the failure to find self-reported and longer-term intervention effects was not the result of problems with implementation.

Indicated programs

Many prevention programs have targeted children and adolescents with increased but subthreshold depression symptoms. This approach is often used in nonschool settings, such as primary care clinics,[56] but is also used in schools. Two school-based programs implemented using an indicated approach are described here.

The Feelings Club Manassis and colleagues[57] tested a 12-session after-school group cognitive behavioral intervention known as The Feelings Club. The program was adapted from the Coping Bear curriculum for child anxiety disorders[58,59] and emphasizes cognitive restructuring techniques for improving negative affect. Participants were 148 children in grades 3 to 6 across 26 schools in a Canadian city. Participants all screened positive for internalizing symptoms and consented to participation; they were randomized either to the intervention or to an after-school activity program of equivalent length. Children's internalizing symptoms improved in both study conditions, with no significant group differences identified, suggesting that the control group activities may also have been beneficial for students. A strength of the study was the use of an active control group, which is a rigorous design that makes it more difficult to demonstrate significant intervention effects.

Personal Growth Class The Personal Growth Class (PGC) is a school-based indicated intervention designed to reduce depressive symptoms and suicide risk in adolescents showing signs and symptoms of risk for suicidal behavior. Program content is shaped by theories of strain, social learning, social control, and social support. Core intervention components include training in social support and life skills. Thompson and colleagues[60] conducted a 3-armed randomized controlled trial with a sample of 106 high school students who screened positive for risk of suicidal behavior. The study compared 1 semester of PGC versus 2 semesters of PGC versus a no-intervention control group.[60] Both intervention groups showed reduced depressive symptoms and reduced suicide risk compared with the control group; some additional benefits were evident for students in the 2-semester condition.

Family-based Approaches

Children and adolescents of depressed parents are 3 to 4 times more likely to develop MDD than their counterparts with nondepressed parents.[61] Interventions targeting children and adolescents of depressed parents have been a focus of intervention research given the potential public health impact of reaching this at-risk population. One of the earliest preventive interventions targeting children and adolescents of depressed parents was conducted by Clarke and colleagues.[62] Adolescents aged 13 to 18 years who had subthreshold depressive symptoms and a parent with MDD received a 16-session cognitive behavioral intervention focused on cognitive restructuring, interpersonal problem solving, and effective communication skills. Adolescents receiving the intervention showed significantly lower rates of MDD at a 12-month follow-up compared with adolescents not receiving the intervention. A larger-scale replication of the trial by Clarke and colleagues,[62] conducted by Garber and colleagues[63] across 4 sites, found significant reductions in participants' depressive symptoms and significantly lower rates of MDD at a 9-month follow-up compared with adolescents not receiving the cognitive behavioral intervention.

Although some family-based interventions, including those described earlier, focus on intervening with children of depressed parents,[62–65] other programs have intervened with both children of depressed parents and the parents themselves. Beardslee and colleagues[66] intervened with 93 families in which a parent had a mood disorder, delivering program components to parents and their children, aged 9 to 15 years. One-third of families participated in the lecture study arm in which parents attended 2 separate meetings without their children, whereas two-thirds of families participated in the clinician study arm consisting of 6 to 11 sessions that included separate meetings with parents and children, family meetings, and refresher meetings. In both intervention conditions, parents were provided with information about mood disorders, skills helpful in communicating with their children, and strategies for promoting discussion with their children about the effects of parental depression. Results indicated that both interventions led to children's increased understanding of parental depression and decreased internalizing symptoms. Compas and colleagues'[67] Family Group Cognitive Behavioral intervention teaches parenting skills to parents with a history of depression and also teaches their children (aged 9–15 years) coping techniques to deal with the stress associated with their parents' depression. A randomized controlled trial found that the intervention was successful in reducing children's and parents' depressive symptoms at a 12-month follow-up.[67] Positive intervention effects were also found on some measures of child mental health at 18-month and 24-month follow-ups, and more than twice as many intervention children versus control children had experienced an episode of major depression by the 24-month follow-up.[68]

Other Settings and Delivery Modalities

Although most depression prevention interventions for children and adolescents still occur in school-based settings, in part because of the ability to recruit study participants, a growing number of interventions have been tested in other settings and through various delivery modalities. With the growing availability and use of Internet and computer technologies, several interventions have attempted to reach children and adolescents via these modalities. A systematic review of Internet and computerized interventions[69] found that computerized cognitive behavioral interventions led to reductions in depressive symptoms among adolescents and young adults (aged 12–25 years), but not younger children (aged 5–11 years). Other types of computerized interventions that focused on attention bias modification and cognitive bias modification of interpretations did not show evidence of efficacy in reducing or preventing depression. Van Voorhees and colleagues used an Internet-based intervention coupled with either motivational interviewing or brief advice provided by a primary care physician to adolescents recruited from primary care practices and found that both intervention arms resulted in decreases in depressive symptoms through a 1-year follow-up.[70] Other settings in which depression prevention interventions have been conducted include primary care,[56] juvenile detention centers,[71] and employment training programs.[72]

DISCUSSION

Several recent systematic reviews and meta-analyses have concluded that there is evidence for beneficial effects of preventive interventions for depression in children and adolescents.[73–76] Effect sizes are generally small but are consistent with, or larger than, the size of effects obtained for preventive interventions to prevent youth substance abuse, human immunodeficiency virus, eating disorders, and obesity.[76]

Merry and colleagues[73] also noted as "very encouraging" their calculation that the reduction in postintervention depression risk is equivalent to a number needed to treat (NNT; the sample size required in order to affect 1 individual) of 11 individuals (confidence interval, 7–20). Moreover, even small effects can translate into substantive benefits over time or across large populations. This section of the article discusses several aspects of the empirical findings to date and suggests directions for future research.

Universal Versus Targeted Prevention Approaches

Prior meta-analyses concluded that selective and indicated prevention strategies were more effective than universal approaches.[76,77] Researchers suggested that targeting youth with subsyndromal symptoms may be more feasible from a resource standpoint than intervening with a larger, nonsymptomatic group given that many young participants in a universal prevention program never develop depressive symptoms or disorder, and extremely large samples may be needed to obtain statistically significant effects.[77] However, a more recent meta-analysis that included a larger number of studies concluded that both universal and targeted prevention programs reduced depressive episodes and depressive symptoms at posttest and 12-month follow-up.[73]

The finding that universal prevention is effective is an encouraging development, because universal programs have several advantages, including the ability to reach at-risk young people who may not be identified by targeting a given risk factor or administering a particular screening instrument. Universal prevention strategies are particularly well suited for schools, where there are often logistical barriers to mental health screening. There is a particular need for universal interventions to promote protective factors in schools serving low-income communities, given these students' high level of trauma exposure, emotional symptoms, and academic challenges.[34] For instance, in a study of elementary schools serving impoverished communities (n = 1099 students), 56% of students were identified as having mental health needs.[78] The public education system is under-resourced and ill equipped to address this level of need using pull-out models, such as indicated programs.[34,78] Moreover, pull-out approaches may not embed intervention models sufficiently within the school ecology to shape school climate.[34] Universal programs that can be integrated with school practices are a resource-efficient and logical prevention approach for a population of young people at very high risk for poor outcomes.[34]

Prevention of Depressive Symptoms Versus Major Depressive Disorder

Most studies have assessed reduction in self-reported depressive symptoms, rather than prevention of MDD incidence, as an outcome of prevention trials. The additional time and expense required for administration of structured clinical interviews makes it difficult to routinely incorporate them into prevention studies, particularly those with large sample sizes. As a result, although there is mounting evidence that some prevention programs prevent MDD incidence,[20,73,76] clinicians must be cautious and not assume that findings regarding depressive symptom reductions automatically translate into prevention of incidence of depressive disorder. Some prevention researchers[77] have additionally argued that reductions in depressive symptoms relative to a lack of change in the control group should be viewed as a treatment rather than a prevention effect; by contrast, prevention should signify symptom reduction or lack of change in the intervention group relative to an increase in the control group. A further complication is that some young people enrolled in prevention trials have had prior episodes of depression; for these participants, intervention effects are perhaps most accurately conceptualized as relapse prevention.[73] Despite these challenges in categorizing prevention, it is clear that young people can benefit substantively from programs that reduce current depressive symptoms and provide mood management strategies that increase long-term resilience against stress.

Moderators of Intervention Effects

Understanding moderators of intervention effects is key to effectively disseminating and implementing prevention programs. Potential moderators (ie, prevention type, depression outcome) were discussed earlier. There is additional heterogeneity per the current literature, including variability in intervention content and length, settings, delivery modalities, and measurement. This diversity makes it more difficult to draw general conclusions about intervention efficacy and suggests that more nuanced evaluation of moderators may be beneficial in identifying the most promising interventions, study designs, and target populations.

Some individual studies have evaluated hypothesized moderators. For instance, some universal prevention programs have examined intervention outcomes by high-risk versus low-risk participant status based on participants' initial symptom levels.[45] Meta-analysis is also a valuable tool for understanding potential moderators, including gender, intervention content, and intervention delivery. Although some earlier reviews found evidence that depression prevention programs were more effective for girls than for boys,[76,77] the most recent Cochrane Review concluded that depression prevention effects did not differ by gender.[73] Program content may also modify outcomes, with some evidence for the efficacy of cognitive behavioral approaches.[73] Stice and colleagues[76] reported that shorter prevention programs were more efficacious than longer programs; by contrast, Horowitz and Garber[77] and Merry and colleagues[73] did not find a significant effect for program length across all programs, although Merry and colleagues[73] reported that, for universal programs only, offering 8 or more sessions was superior to fewer sessions. Intervention delivery modality has also been explored as a possible moderator of prevention effects, with some evidence for stronger effect sizes when interventions were implemented by mental health professionals rather than teachers.[75,76] Fewer Internet-based programs have been tested, but future research should compare Internet-based delivery with more traditional delivery models.

Study Limitations

The evidence base for depression prevention for children and adolescents is growing rapidly, increasing confidence in the consistency and nature of prevention effects. However, many studies have methodological flaws that limit to some extent the conclusions that can be drawn about intervention effects. Perhaps the most significant issue is that few studies have included active (placebo) comparison groups that control for time, attention from adults, and other nonspecific benefits to which intervention participants are exposed. Not surprisingly, studies that included attention control groups tended to report attenuated intervention effects relative to those that do not.[75] However, the consistency of effects across studies and the fact that many show continued effects at 6, 9, and even 12 months after the intervention mitigate to some extent concerns about the lack of attention control groups.[73] In addition, studies have rarely used allocation concealment (blinding of participants and assessment staff as to study condition), which is an important criterion for high-quality randomized controlled trials.[73] Allocation concealment for participants is challenging in studies without an attention control condition because it is obvious which group is receiving the intervention. However, studies with an attention control condition (ie, nutrition program) are offering 2 potentially beneficial options to participants and may be able to withhold information about which program is being evaluated as the intervention condition. Many studies have also not included long-term follow-up assessments, making it more difficult to determine the extent to which prevention effects persist over time. Follow-ups are also important for identifying so-called sleeper effects, because some studies have reported increased efficacy of depression prevention interventions at follow-up.[79] Many studies in the current literature are also hampered by small sample sizes, which reduce the power to detect effects and to examine potential moderators.

Future Directions

Future research should target current design limitations, incorporating attention control conditions, allocation concealment, large sample sizes, tests of moderation, and long-term follow-up assessments whenever possible. Clinicians should identify and build on those programs with the strongest evidence base, in order to effectively disseminate them on a broader scale. Collection of data on cost and cost-effectiveness is critical with respect to informing dissemination and scale-up efforts and should be systematically gathered. Prevention programs that can be effectively implemented by non–mental health professionals, such as teachers, will greatly advance the potential to deliver interventions cost-effectively on a large scale. Developing effective ways to train and support teachers and other lay people in serving as intervention facilitators is an important area for further research.

Almost all depression prevention programs incorporate cognitive behavior therapy (CBT) elements (eg, cognitive restructuring), but there are few empirical evaluations about which active ingredients may be most successful across prevention programs. It is helpful for studies to specify intervention content, as well as hypothesized core components and mechanisms, in order to facilitate comparisons across programs and better understanding of the mechanisms by which programs may effect change. Individual studies should also be designed with sufficient power to test hypothesized mediation pathways. Programs using non-CBT intervention strategies, including interpersonal therapy (IPT),[80] mindfulness-based strategies,[81,82] and exercise,[83] have shown initial promise and merit further study and comparison with cognitive behavioral interventions. Moreover, it is important to evaluate whether different intervention approaches have different levels of fit as a function of the prevention approach used (universal, selective, indicated) and target population served. For instance, exercise-based programs may be better suited than IPT to universal implementation, and participant age, gender, cultural identity, or socioeconomic status may shape intervention preferences.

Hybrid or stepped-care approaches that offer universal prevention programs, followed by more targeted interventions for youth who do not respond to the initial program, merit further study. These models may also benefit from a combination of intervention delivery methods, with universal components offered by non–mental health professionals, such as teachers, and indicated components for nonresponders offered by trained personnel, such as school counselors. Internet-delivered content and other technology-based approaches (eg, text message reminders, apps) should also be explored as ways to augment or enhance intervention content (**Box 2**).

Box 2
Directions for future research

- Conduct randomized controlled studies with more rigorous design features:
  ○ Larger sample sizes
  ○ Attention control conditions
  ○ Allocation concealment for participants and assessment staff
  ○ Follow-up assessments over longer time periods ($\geq$12 months)
  ○ Cost and cost-benefit analyses
- Develop methods for promoting effective delivery by non–mental health professionals (eg, teachers)
- Test theory-based mechanisms of intervention effects
- Evaluate stepped-care approaches and use of multiple intervention delivery modalities
- Lay the groundwork for large-scale effectiveness trials to evaluate dissemination and implementation

---

SUMMARY

Prevention science has made great progress since the Institute of Medicine advocated the study of prevention of mental disorders in 1994. The literature suggests that depression prevention in children and adolescents is feasible and shows promising evidence for efficacy. The next phase is large-scale dissemination and implementation of evidence-based depression prevention interventions within systems that serve young people.

REFERENCES

1. Avenevoli S, Swendson J, He J, et al. Major depression in the National Comorbidity Survey–Adolescent Supplement: prevalence, correlates, and treatment. J Am Acad Child Adolesc Psychiatry 2015;54(1):37–44.e2.
2. Kessler RC, Walters EE. Epidemiology of DSM-III-R major depression and minor depression among adolescents and young adults in the National Comorbidity Study. Depress Anxiety 1998;7:3–14.
3. Kessler RC, Wai CT, Demler O, et al. Prevalence, severity, and comorbidity of 12-month DSM-IV disorders in the National Comorbidity Survey Replication. Arch Gen Psychiatry 2005;62:617–27.
4. Klein DN, Shankman SA, Lewinsohn PM, et al. Subthreshold depressive disorder in adolescents: Predictors of escalation to full-syndrome depressive disorders. J Am Acad Child Adolesc Psychiatry 2009;48:703–10.
5. Brent DA, Weersing VR. Depressive disorders in childhood and adolescence. In: Rutter M, Bishop B, Pine D, et al, editors. Rutters' child and adolescent psychiatry. Oxford (United Kingdom): Blackwell Publishing; 2008. p. 587–613.
6. Costello EJ, Pine DS, Hammen C, et al. Development and natural history of mood disorders. Biol Psychiatry 2002;52:529–42.
7. Shankman SA, Lewinsohn PM, Klein DN, et al. Subthreshold conditions as precursors for full syndrome disorders: a 15-year longitudinal study of multiple diagnostic classes. J Child Psychol Psychiatry 2009;50:1485–94.
8. Munoz RF, Mrazek PJ, Haggerty RJ. Institute of Medicine report on prevention of mental disorders: summary and commentary. Am Psychol 1996;51: 1116–22.

9. Casacalenda N, Perry JC, Looper K. Remission in major depressive disorder: a comparison of pharmacotherapy, psychotherapy, and control conditions. Am J Psychiatry 2002;159(8):1354–60.

10. Kakuma R, Minas H, van Ginneken N, et al. Human resources for mental health care: current situation and strategies for action. Lancet 2011;378(9803).1654–63.

11. Mojtabai R, Olfson M, Sampson NA, et al. Barriers to mental health treatment: results from the National Comorbidity Survey Replication (NCS-R). Psychol Med 2011;41(8):1751–61.

12. Panel DG. Depression in primary care: Vol 2. Treatment of major depression. Rockville (MD): Agency for Health Care Policy and Research; 1993.

13. Andrews G, Wilkinson DD. The prevention of mental disorders in young people. Med J Aust 2002;177:S97–100.

14. Andrews G, Issakidis C, Sanderson K, et al. Utilising survey data to inform public policy: comparison of the cost-effectiveness of treatment of ten mental disorders. Br J Psychiatry 2004;184:526–33.

15. Moussavi S, Chatterji S, Verdes E, et al. Depression, chronic diseases, and decrements in health: results from the World Health Surveys. Lancet 2007;370(9590): 8–14.

16. Davis LL, Uezeto A, Newell JM, et al. Major depression and comorbid substance use disorders. Curr Opin Psychiatry 2008;21(1):14–8.

17. Sartorius N, Ustun TB, Lecrubier Y, et al. Depression comorbid with anxiety: results from the WHO study on psychological disorders in primary health care. Br J Psychiatry Suppl 1996;30:38–43.

18. Panel DG. Depression in primary care: detection, diagnosis, and treatment: quick reference guide for clinicians. Rockville (MD): Agency for Health Care Policy and Research; 1993.

19. Judd LL. The clinical course of unipolar major depressive disorders. Arch Gen Psychiatry 1997;54:989–91.

20. Cuijpers P, van Straten A, Smit F, et al. Preventing the onset of depressive disorders: a meta-analytic review of psychological interventions. Am J Psychiatry 2008;165:1272–80.

21. Benefits and costs of prevention and early intervention programs for youth, technical appendix. Washington State Institute for Public Policy. 2004. Available at: http://wsipp.wa.gov/rptfiles/04-07-3901a.pdf. Accessed September 5, 2015.

22. Anderson P, Chisholm D, Fuhr DC. Effectiveness and cost-effectiveness of policies and programmes to reduce the harm caused by alcohol. Lancet 2009; 373:2234–46.

23. Zechmeister I, Kilian R, McDaid D. Is it worth investing in mental health promotion and prevention of mental illness? A systematic review of the evidence from economic evaluations. BMC Public Health 2008;8:20.

24. National Research Council, Institute of Medicine. Preventing mental, emotional, and behavioral disorders among young people: progress and possibilities. Washington, DC: The National Academies Press; 2009.

25. Rose G. The strategy of preventive medicine. Oxford (United Kingdom): Oxford University Press; 1992.

26. Kellam SG, Koretz D, Moscicki EK. Core elements of developmental epidemiologically based prevention research. Am J Community Psychol 1999;27(4):463–82.

27. Flay BR, Biglan A, Boruch RF, et al. Standards of evidence: criteria for efficacy, effectiveness, and dissemination. Prev Sci 2005;6:151–75.

28. Ialongo NS, Kellam SG, Poduska JM. A developmental framework for clinical child and pediatric psychology research. In: Drotar D, editor. Handbook of

research in pediatric and clinical child psychiatry: practical strategies and methods. New York: Kluwer Academic/Plenum Publishers; 2000. p. 3–19.

29. Gladstone TRG, Beardslee WR, O'Connor EE. The prevention of adolescent depression. Psychiatr Clin North Am 2011;34:35–52.

30. N.R.C., I.O.M.. The etiology of depression. Depression in parents, parenting, and children. Washington, DC: National Academies Press; 2009. p. 73–118.

31. Joorman J, Eugene F, Gotlib IH. Parental depression: Impact on offspring and mechanisms underlying transmission of risk. In: Nolen-Hoeksems S, Hilt LM, editors. Handbook of depression in adolescence. New York: Taylor & Francis Group; 2009. p. 441–72.

32. Mrazek PJ, Haggerty RJ. Reducing risks for mental disorders: frontiers for preventive intervention research. Washington, DC: National Academy Press; 1994.

33. Adelman HS, Taylor L. Mental health in schools: engaging learners, preventing problems, and improving schools. Thousand Oaks (CA): Corwin Press; 2010.

34. Atkins MS, Hoagwood KE, Kutash K, et al. Toward the integration of education and mental health in schools. Adm Policy Ment Health 2010;37:40–7.

35. Domitrovich CE, Bradshaw CP, Greenberg MT, et al. Integrated models of school-based prevention: logic and theory. Psychol Sch 2010;47:71–88.

36. Masten AS. Commentary: developmental psychopathology as a unifying context for mental health and education models, research, and practice in schools. Sch Psychol Rev 2003;32(2):169–73.

37. Shochet I, Holland D, Whitefield K. Resourceful adolescent program: group leader's manual. Brisbane (Australia): Griffith University; 1997.

38. Merry S, McDowell H, Wild CJ, et al. A randomized placebo-controlled trial of a school-based depression prevention program. J Am Acad Child Adolesc Psychiatry 2004;43(5):538–47.

39. Shochet IM, Dadds MR, Holland D, et al. The efficacy of a universal school-based program to prevent adolescent depression. J Clin Child Psychol 2001;30(3):303–15.

40. Stallard P, Buck R. Preventing depression and promoting resilience: feasibility study of a school-based cognitive-behavioural intervention. Br J Psychiatry 2013;202:S18–23.

41. Sawyer MG, Pfeiffer S, Spence SH, et al. School-based prevention of depression: a randomised controlled study of the beyondblue schools research initiative. J Child Psychol Psychiatry 2010;51(2):199–209.

42. Sawyer MG, Harchak TF, Spence SH, et al. School-based prevention of depression: a 2-year follow-up of a randomized controlled trial of the beyondblue schools research initiative. J Adolesc Health 2010;47(3):297–304.

43. Beck AT, Rush AJ, Shaw BF, et al. Cognitive therapy of depression. New York: The Guilford Press; 1979.

44. D'Zurilla TJ, Nezu A. A study of the generation-of-alternatives process in social problem solving. Cognit Ther Res 1980;4:67–72.

45. Spence SH, Sheffield JK, Donovan CL. Preventing adolescent depression: an evaluation of the Problem Solving for Life program. J Consult Clin Psychol 2003;71(1):3–13.

46. Spence SH, Sheffield JK, Donovan CL. Long-term outcome of a school-based, universal approach to prevention of depression in adolescents. J Consult Clin Psychol 2005;73(1):160–7.

47. Brunwasser SM, Gilham JE, Kim ES. A meta-analytic review of the Penn Resiliency Program's effect on depressive symptoms. J Consult Clin Psychol 2009; 77(6):1042–54.

48. Cardemil EV, Reivich KJ, Seligman ME. The prevention of depressive symptoms in low-income minority middle school students. Prev Treat 2002. [Epub ahead of print].

49. Cardemil EV, Reivich KJ, Beevers CG, et al. The prevention of depressive symptoms in low-income, minority children: two-year follow-up. Behav Res Ther 2007; 45:313–27.

50. Vega WA, Rumbaut RG. Ethnic minorities and mental health. Annu Rev Sociol 1991;17:351–83.

51. Bruce ML, Takeuchi DT, Leaf PJ. Poverty and psychiatric status: longitudinal evidence from the epidemiologic catchment area study. Arch Gen Psychiatry 1991; 48:470–4.

52. Vega WA, Kolody B, Aguilar-Gaxiola S, et al. Lifetime prevalence of DSM-III-R psychiatric diagnoses among urban and rural Mexican Americans in California. Arch Gen Psychiatry 1998;55:771–8.

53. Roberts C, Ballantyne F, van der Klift P. Aussie optimism. Social life skills. Teacher resource. Perth (Australia): Curtin University of Technology; 2003.

54. Roberts R, Roberts C, Cosgrove S, et al. Aussie optimism. Optimistic thinking skills. Teacher resource. Perth (Australia): Curtin University of Technology; 2003.

55. Roberts CM, Kane R, Bishop B, et al. The prevention of anxiety and depression in children from disadvantaged schools. Behav Res Ther 2010;48:68–73.

56. Gilham JE, Hamilton J, Freres DR, et al. Preventing depression among early adolescents in the primary care setting: a randomized controlled trial of the Penn Resiliency Program. J Abnorm Child Psychol 2006;34:203–19.

57. Manassis K, Wilansky-Traynor P, Farzan N, et al. The feelings club: randomized controlled evaluation of school-based CBT for anxious or depressive symptoms. Depress Anxiety 2010;27:945–52.

58. Manassis K, Mendleowitz S, Scapillato D, et al. Group and individual cognitive behavior therapy for childhood anxiety disorders: a randomized trial. J Am Acad Child Adolesc Psychiatry 2002;41.1423–30.

59. Mendleowitz S, Manassis K, Bradley S, et al. Cognitive behavioral group treatments in childhood anxiety disorders: the role of parental involvement. J Am Acad Child Adolesc Psychiatry 1999;38:1223–9.

60. Thompson EA, Eggert LL, Hertig JR. Mediating effects of an indicated prevention program for reducing youth depression and suicide risk behaviors. Suicide Life Threat Behav 2000;30(3):252–71.

61. Weissman MM, Wickramaratne P, Nomura Y, et al. Offspring of depressed parents: 20 years later. Am J Psychiatry 2006;163(6):1001–8.

62. Clarke GN, Hornbrook M, Lynch F, et al. A randomized trial of a group cognitive intervention for preventing depression in adolescent offspring of depressed parents. Arch Gen Psychiatry 2001;58:1127–34.

63. Garber J, Clarke GN, Weersing VR, et al. Prevention of depression in at-risk adolescents: a randomized controlled trial. J Am Med Assoc 2009;301:2215–24.

64. Beardslee WR, Brent DA, Weersing VR, et al. Prevention of depression in at-risk adolescents: longer-term effects. JAMA Psychiatry 2013;70(11):1161–70.

65. Punamaki RL, Paavonen J, Toikka S, et al. Effectiveness of preventive family intervention in improving cognitive attributions among children of depressed parents: a randomized study. J Fam Psychol 2013;27:683–90.

66. Beardslee WR, Gladstone TRG, Wright EJ, et al. A family-based approach to the prevention of depressive symptoms in children at risk: evidence of parental and child change. Pediatrics 2003;112:119–31.

67. Compas BE, Forehand R, Keller G, et al. Randomized controlled trial of a family cognitive-behavioral preventive intervention for children of depressed parents. J Consult Clin Psychol 2009;77:1007–20.
68. Compas BE, Forehand R, Thigpen JC, et al. Family group cognitive-behavioral preventive intervention for families of depressed parents: 18- and 24-month outcomes. J Consult Clin Psychol 2011;79(4):488–99.
69. Pennant M, Loucas C, Whittington C, et al. Computerised therapies for anxiety and depression in children and young people: a systematic review and meta-analysis. Behav Res Ther 2015;67:1–18.
70. Saulsberry A, Marko-Holquin M, Blomeke K, et al. Randomized clinical trial of a primary-care internet-based intervention to prevent adolescent depression: one-year outcomes. J Can Acad Child Adolesc Psychiatry 2013;22(2):106–17.
71. MacMahon JF, Gross RT. Physical and psychological effects of aerobic exercise in delinquent adolescents males. Am J Dis Child 1988;142:1361–6.
72. Tandon SD, Latimore AD, Clay E, et al. Depression outcomes associated with an intervention implemented in employment training programs for low-income adolescents and young adults. JAMA Psychiatry 2015;72(1):31–9.
73. Merry SN, Hetrick SE, Cox GR, et al. Psychological and educational interventions for preventing depression in children and adolescents. Cochrane Database Syst Rev 2011;(12):CD003380.
74. Corrieri S, Heider D, Conrad IB, et al. School-based prevention programs for depression and anxiety in adolescence: a systematic review. Health Promot Internation 2013;29(3):427–41.
75. Calear AL, Christensen H. Systematic review of school-based prevention and early intervention programs for depression. J Adolesc 2010;33:429–38.
76. Stice E, Shaw H, Bohon C, et al. A meta-analytic review of depression prevention programs for children and adolescents: factors that predict magnitude of intervention effects. J Consult Clin Psychol 2009;77(3):486–503.
77. Horowitz JL, Garber J. The prevention of depressive symptoms in children and adolescents: a meta-analytic review. J Consult Clin Psychol 2006;74(3):401–15.
78. Baker JA, Kamphaus RW, Horne AM, et al. Evidence for population-based perspectives on children's behavioral adjustment and needs for service delivery in schools. Sch Psychol Rev 2006;35(1):31–46.
79. Gillham JE, Shatte AJ, Reivich KJ. Needed for prevention research: long-term follow up and the evaluation of mediators, moderators, and lay providers. Prev Treat 2001. [Epub ahead of print].
80. Young JF, Mufson L, Davies M. Efficacy of interpersonal psychotherapy adolescent skills training: an indicated preventive intervention for depression. J Child Psychol Psychiatry 2006;47(12):1254–62.
81. Mendelson T, Tandon SD, O'Brennan L, et al. Brief report: moving prevention into schools: the impact of a trauma-informed school-based intervention. J Adolesc 2015;43:142–7.
82. Zenner C, Herrnleben-Kurz S, Walach H. Mindfulness-based interventions in schools–a systematic review and meta-analysis. Front Psychol 2014;5:603.
83. Brown HE, Pearson N, Braithewaite RE, et al. Physical activity interventions and depression in children and adolescents: a systematic review and meta-analysis. Sports Med 2013;43:195–206.

Suicide Prevention Strategies for Improving Population Health

Holly C. Wilcox, PhD[a,b,*], Peter A. Wyman, PhD[c]

KEYWORDS

• Suicide • Attempted suicide • Public health • Prevention and control

KEY POINTS

• Suicide is the second leading cause of death among 15 to 19 year olds.
• Suicide prevention efforts have relied heavily on gatekeeper training programs, but this approach alone will not be successful.
• Coordinated interventions are needed at all levels (primary, secondary, and tertiary).

OVERVIEW

Annual suicide rates among those 10-24 years old have increased since 2008 in the United States.[1] In 2014, suicide was the second leading cause of death among those ages 15 to 19.[1] Over 1 million high school students are treated by a nurse or doctor annually for a suicide attempt.[2]

In 2014, the National Action Alliance for Suicide Prevention Research Prioritization Task Force prioritized the prevention of "the emergence of suicidal behavior by

Funding Sources: Dr H.C. Wilcox: National Institute of Mental Health (NIMH [R01MH095855]), American Foundation for Suicide Prevention (AFSP [LSRG-1-010-13]), Agency for Healthcare Research and Quality (AHRQ [Contract No. 290-2012-000007I]) and Substance Abuse and Mental Health Services Administration (U79SM061751). Dr P.A. Wyman: National Institute on Mental Health (NIMH), Department of Defense.
Conflict of Interest: Nil.
[a] Department of Psychiatry & Behavioral Sciences, Johns Hopkins University School of Medicine, 550 North Broadway, Room 921, Baltimore, MD 21287, USA; [b] Department of Mental Health, Johns Hopkins Bloomberg School of Public Health, 550 North Broadway, Room 921, Baltimore, MD 21287, USA; [c] Department of Psychiatry, University of Rochester School of Medicine and Dentistry, University of Rochester Medical Center, 300 Crittenden Boulevard, Rochester, NY 14642, USA
* Corresponding author. Johns Hopkins University, 550 North Broadway, Room 921, Baltimore, MD 21287.
E-mail address: hwilcox1@jhmi.edu

Child Adolesc Psychiatric Clin N Am 25 (2016) 219–233
http://dx.doi.org/10.1016/j.chc.2015.12.003
1056-4993/16/$ – see front matter © 2016 Elsevier Inc. All rights reserved.

developing and delivering the most effective prevention programs to build resilience and reduce risk in broad-based populations."[3]

DEFINITIONS

Because the definitions of suicidal behavior vary greatly, it is challenging to combine or compare the results of studies.[4] Consistent definitions would allow researchers to better estimate the scope of the problem, identify high-risk groups, and monitor the effects of prevention programs and policies. Until 1996, there was no standard nomenclature (common vocabulary) for suicide-related behaviors. Multiple terms are used in the literature to describe suicide-related behaviors (eg, self-destructive behavior, suicide, suicide attempt, completed suicide, suicide gesture, suicide acts, self-directed violence, deliberate self-harm, parasuicide [suicide attempt that does not result in death], self-inflicted injury, intrapersonal violence, and self-mutilation).

These terms vary in usage geographically and can differ by level of lethality and suicide intent. To facilitate communication and comparison of data, definitions were proposed by O'Carroll and colleagues[5] (1996) with a revision proposed in 2007 by Silverman and colleagues.[6] The extent to which these recommended definitions are followed is unclear. The current definitions advocated by the Centers for Disease Control and Prevention[7] are as follows:

- *Suicide:* Death caused by self-directed injurious behavior with an intent to die as a result of the behavior.
- *Suicide attempt:* A nonfatal, self-directed, potentially injurious behavior with an intent to die as a result of the behavior; might not result in injury.
- *Suicidal ideation:* Thinking about, considering, or planning suicide.

THEORETIC FRAMEWORKS AND MODELS

There is no single, widely accepted theoretic framework guiding youth suicide prevention. According to the model from Shaffer and Craft,[8] suicide attempts whether fatal or nonfatal, rarely occur "out of the blue." Within the context of a mood disorder, substance abuse, and/or aggressive traits, suicidal ideation is often preceded by stressful life events such as humiliation, disciplinary crises, trouble with the law or at school, or the loss of a relationship. These stressful life events or crises could be the result of an underlying psychiatric condition. This chain of events, in most instances, does not lead to suicide attempts.

Inhibitory and facilitating factors come into play after the stressful event and the balance between these factors will contribute to either suicide or survival.[8] According to this model, inhibiting factors make suicide less likely and include living in a culture with strong taboo against suicide, having available social support or the presence of others, and having a "slowed down" mental state (ie, psychomotor retardation). Conversely, other factors may facilitate suicide including living in a culture in which taboos about suicide are weak, having ready access to firearms or other methods of suicide, learning of a recent suicide or exposure to publicized suicides, having impulsive-aggressive traits, and being alone (**Fig. 1**). The frontal cortex area of the brain which governs judgment, decision making, and impulse control does not fully mature until around age 25,[9,10] which could explain why some teenagers could appear quick from thought to action in times of perceived crisis.[11]

What is missing from this model are distal factors such as childhood adversity and trauma exposure; genetic and epigenetic influences; the ability to regulate emotion, cognition, and behavior; and the influences of the broader social network.

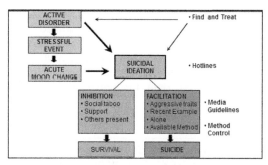

Fig. 1. Factors leading to suicide or survival. (*Adapted from* Shaffer D, Craft L. Methods of adolescent suicide prevention. J Clin Psychiatry 1999;60(Suppl 2):71.)

The most common suicide prevention approach used to date has been to identify and treat individuals already in crisis or with symptoms and disorders linked to suicide via screening in schools, primary care, emergency departments, juvenile justice, child welfare, and other community settings. Among those in crisis or contemplating suicide, hotlines can be used such as the National Suicide Prevention Lifeline. In addition to these 'staples' of suicide prevention, other efforts include limiting physical access to suicide methods (ie, by restricting access to firearms) as well as reducing the cognitive availability of suicide methods (ie, limiting awareness of suicide as an option and knowledge of possible means of suicide which can be achieved via the responsible reporting on suicide by the media).[11]

In summary, suicide is a complex event. Facilitating and inhibitory processes interact to either increase or decrease suicide risk. Many of the risk factors presented herein are not unique to suicide and the potential for suicide increases with the burden of risk. Suicide is rarely the outcome of a single risk factor or event such as bullying. Suicide is preventable and there are opportunities for preventive intervention along multiple points in the complex pathways leading to suicide.

CHALLENGES IN SUICIDE PREVENTION

Many youth suicide prevention programs are listed on the National Registry of Evidence based Programs and Practices, but few have evidence from randomized trials and most target individuals already in crisis. Some challenges suicide prevention scientists encounter are that (1) suicide is a rare outcome so it is challenging to detect an intervention impact on suicide mortality without large studies[12]; (2) misclassification and underreporting of suicide and suicide attempt as outcomes exist owing to stigma and other issues; (3) there is no single, comprehensive national system to document the scope of nonfatal suicide attempts. There are also challenges related to financing and sustaining large-scale, coordinated suicide prevention efforts. Many suicide prevention programs have limited ability to study long-term outcomes under the current funding structure. National, state, and community administrative or surveillance data systems (eg, electronic health records, mortality data, CDC Youth Risk Behavior Surveillance System data) could be linked to existing data from suicide prevention efforts to study the longer term and broader impact of the intervention. However, linking existing suicide prevention program data with data systems has not been done often, possibly owing to associated costs, feasibility of accessing data systems, applicability, and issues of sharing protected health information.

As pointed out by the Data and Surveillance Task Force of the National Action Alliance for Suicide Prevention,[13] the data systems currently used to estimate trends in suicidal behavior were not designed solely to address this subject. In these data systems, questions specific to suicidal behavior are often limited, and the collected data rarely provide the depth of information desired to inform effective prevention and intervention efforts. There is a significant lag (~2–3 years) from when suicides happen until the time when the Centers for Disease Control and Prevention data become available, making it difficult to use these data for prevention approaches informed by surveillance.[13]

Prevention Programs

The goals and target populations of suicide prevention efforts differ by primary, secondary, and tertiary intervention levels. Primary prevention efforts are ideally implemented before young people enter the period of risk for suicide and involve resilience and skills building interventions or policies and legislation to protect individuals (eg, restricting access to firearms). Most existing youth suicide interventions are secondary prevention approaches involving identification of children and adolescents with risk factors for suicide and referring them for assessment and/or treatment. Tertiary suicide prevention approaches are aimed at preventing suicide among suicidal youths. We first review the more common secondary and tertiary prevention approaches, followed by presenting evidence on primary prevention programs. Promising and evidence-based prevention programs are reviewed herein while highlighting prevention principles and implementation strategies.

SECONDARY PREVENTION
Gatekeeper Training

Gatekeeper Training (GKT) programs, currently the most widely used type of youth suicide prevention programming,[14] refer to programs that seek to develop individuals' "knowledge, attitudes and skills to identify (those) at risk, determine levels of risk, and make referrals when necessary."[15] GKT programs typically have 4 main components: (1) increase knowledge about suicide, (2) improve beliefs and attitudes about suicide prevention, (3) decrease reluctance to ask about suicide and persuade suicidal individuals to get help and refer them for help, and (4) enhance self-efficacy to intervene.[16] Sometimes the focus is on practical communication skills, and role play activities are used to practice or reinforce the skills. At least 40 GKT programs exist and they are heterogeneous in terms of content, target audiences, program objectives, training costs, duration (30 minutes to several days), and method of delivery (online or in person). Some programs require awareness of referral resources, institutional policies, and crisis management plans. A variety of individuals who could encounter at-risk youth are trained as gatekeepers, including school or college educators and staff, peer leaders, counseling staff, juvenile justice staff, foster parents, parents or family members, clergy, and health care professionals such as emergency medicine and primary care practitioners. The most common goal of these programs is to encourage gatekeepers to ask directly about suicidal ideation, such as: Are you considering suicide? and Are you thinking of killing yourself? and to link those deemed at risk with mental health professionals.

One of the few randomized trials of GKT tested Question, Persuade, and Refer in 2004 to 2006 in Cobb County, Georgia, in 32 secondary schools with 52,000 students.[17] In this trial, 1.5 hours of GKT was provided for staff, 6 to 8 hours for a counselor in each school, and booster training was provided. Question, Persuade, and Refer increased the knowledge, attitudes, and efficacy of staff; however, increased staff 'communication' with youth about distress only occurred among a small number of staff already engaged in those conversations. Findings from this trial suggested that detecting suicidal students requires adults to be actively engaging with distressed students. The difficulty in detecting suicidal youth outside a close relationship was underscored by results of surveys with students in the same study, which showed that students with a suicide attempt in the past year were less likely to report positive help-seeking attitudes for getting help from an adult and were less likely to believe that their friends or parents will support their seeking help.[17] There is no evidence of effectiveness of GKT, alone without other interventions, in preventing suicidal behaviors[17–19] and, alarmingly, 1 study reported a trend toward an increase in suicidal ideation among those who participated in GKT.[18] Interactive GKT methods seem to be more effective. GKT programs are unlikely to reduce suicide rates without other coordinated, complementary, and effective suicide prevention interventions also in place.

Sources of Strength

Sources of Strength (available at: http://www.sourcesofstrength.org) combines primary and secondary prevention by preparing middle and high school students identified as 'key opinion leaders' to disseminate school-wide healthy norms and practices for coping, and to increase youth–adult connections with ongoing adult mentoring.[20,21] Sources of Strength was developed by Mark LoMurray in collaboration with the North Dakota Adolescent Suicide Prevention Task Force and Department of Health and was named in 2005 a national Field Project Award Winner by the American Public Health Association Epidemiology Section. Sources of Strength as delivered in high schools has 3 phases: school and community preparation, peer leader recruitment and training, and school-wide messaging.

School and community preparation

This first phase includes engagement of the school administration, staff, and community partners; training of adult advisors to prepare them for their role in reinforcing school-wide program concepts; and mentoring student peer leaders in safe suicide prevention messaging.

Peer leader recruitment and training

A standard process is used to nominate and recruit diverse student 'opinion leaders' (15–50 depending on school size). Peer Leaders are trained through a 4-hour interactive workshop led by 1 to 2 certified trainers. A major focus of training is to increase students' knowledge and efficacy to use 'sources of strength' to help adolescents cope with psychosocial challenges (eg, conflict with parents, relationship breakups) and emotions (eg, anger, depression, and anxiety). The focus of training is to prepare peer leaders to complete tasks designed to spread information and norms about sources of strength throughout their school.

School-wide messaging phase

With close adult advisor supervision, peer leaders develop recommended prevention activities so that they can introduce their friends and other students to using Sources of Strength, including trusted adults, and overcoming barriers to engaging help for oneself and friends who may be distressed.

Sources of Strength intervention conceptual model Sources of Strength is intended to strengthen social–ecological and individual protective factors,[21] including connectedness with adults, family, and school, and social integration with competent peers.[22] Protective effects from connectedness include meeting needs for belonging,[23] increasing psychological well-being, reducing perceptions of threat from stressors,[24] and teaching positive coping strategies for managing distress through engaging support.[25,26] The delivery model is congruent with the diffusion of innovations theory[27] and Valente's social network thresholds model,[28] which point to the importance of interpersonal persuasion of trusted others in the decision to adopt new behaviors. For higher risk youth, increased exposure to positive coping norms is intended to reduce the likelihood of suicidal ideation progressing to attempts or death by suicide. For lower risk youth, these protective processes are intended to enhance coping and reduce the likelihood of entering a trajectory that includes suicidal behavior.

Research documenting Sources of Strength impact A cluster randomized controlled trial in 18 schools with 465 peer leaders and 2700 students showed that 4 months of the Sources of Strength intervention enhanced protective factors associated with reducing suicide at a school population level.[21] After training and 4 months of messaging, trained peer leaders, compared with those in control schools, gained in adaptive norms regarding suicide, connectedness to adults, and use of resources for coping, with standardized effect sizes ranging from 0.22 to 0.75. Trained peer leaders in larger schools were 4 times more likely as untrained peer leaders in control schools to refer a suicidal friend to an adult. Among students in the population, 4 months of Sources of Strength messaging had medium-sized effects on increasing help seeking acceptance (effective size (ES) = 0.58) and modifying student expectations that adults in their schools will help suicidal peers (ES = 0.63). The greatest increase in norms from baseline to follow-up was for suicidal youth. Thus, Sources of Strength had stronger effects on those adolescents most at risk for suicide. An ongoing National Institute of Mental Health-funded randomized trial with 40 high schools and 14,000 students is testing the impact of the intervention on reducing self-reported suicide attempts.

Challenges to implementing Sources of Strength include recruiting peer leaders, especially those with 'reach' to students at higher risk of suicide, including students who are socially isolated from peer groups.[21] In a current ongoing trial, schools with reduced peer leader diversity and lower retention of peer leaders had lower implementation success in meeting key first-year milestones of disseminating Sources of Strength concepts to the broader school population and increasing student-to-student conversation about using coping resources.[23]

Signs of Suicide

Signs of Suicide is an evidence-based secondary school-based suicide prevention program that includes screening and an educational curriculum focused on how to cope with depression and common adolescent life challenges, including getting help for self or others. Three randomized trials have shown short-term decreases in self-reported suicide attempts among students receiving Signs of Suicide using posttest assessments after 3 months.[29–31] Decreased suicide attempts were not owing to self-reported increased help seeking, suggesting that Signs of Suicide may be reducing suicidal behavior through another mechanism. This program has also been implemented with middle school students.[32]

Interactive Screening Program

As is outlined by Haas and colleagues,[33] the American Foundation for Suicide Prevention has developed and disseminated to colleges and other settings a screening program that identifies individuals at risk for suicide via an email invitation offering them the opportunity to participate in an online, web-based screening. The ISP provides an anonymous, web-based method of outreach that starts with a brief, confidential online Stress and Depression Questionnaire. Each university or other organization decides whom to target through the program, and these individuals receive an email invitation to engage in ISP.

The questionnaire incorporates the Patient Health Questionnaire-9, a 9-item standardized depression screening scale that has been validated in 2 large, multisite studies and found to be strongly predictive of major depressive disorder.[34,35] In addition to the depression items, the Stress and Depression Questionnaire contains questions about suicidal ideation and attempts, problems related to depression such as anger and anxiety, alcohol and drug abuse, and eating disorder symptoms. The questionnaire contains approximately 35 questions and normally takes less than 10 minutes to complete.

At the end of the questionnaire, participants are asked to provide an email address so that they can be notified when a counselor has prepared a personalized response and posted it to their attention on the program website. Participants are assured that their email address will be encrypted into the computer system to protect their identity, and will not be made available to anyone, including the counselor who will be responding to them.

After the participant submits the questionnaire, it is analyzed by computer and, based on specific answers, the participant is classified into one of 4 tiers; 1A, 1B, 2, or 3, with 1A suggesting highest risk and 3 lowest risk. The computer system then generates an email to the counselor, which indicates the participant's tier level and provides a link to the participant's record on the secure website.

On the website page where the counselor's response is posted, a "Dialogue" button provides direct access to a page where the participant can send a message to the counselor. Participants may exchange messages with the counselor on an unlimited basis, although the counselor will continue to urge participants with significant problems to arrange an in-person meeting. The dialogues with the counselor play a critical role in the process of encouraging the participant to seek help by facilitating the resolution of barriers to treatment. The dialogues offer an opportunity for the participant to begin to develop a trusting relationship with the counselor, which increases the likelihood that they will ultimately accept the counselor's invitation for a face-to-face meeting.

Screening in Pediatric Medical Settings

Most mental health problems never reach mental health services owing to problems with detection, stigma, and access to care. There is a strong need to integrate behavioral health services into primary and secondary care settings. Patients who present to the emergency department with suicidal thoughts and behaviors are at increased risk for suicide. Suicide risk screening in pediatric emergency departments comply with the Joint Commission National Patient Safety Goals (NPSG.15.01.01), requiring behavioral health care organizations, psychiatric hospitals, and general hospitals treating individuals for emotional or behavioral disorders to identify individuals at risk for suicide. The Ask Suicide Screening Questions instrument[36] is in the public domain and is easy to administer and score. This instrument could be used for universal (all patients) or indicated (only those with a psychiatric presenting complaint) screening in emergency departments. Parent education and restricting access to lethal means have to also be addressed in these settings.[37]

Up to 66% of patients who die by suicide see their primary care doctor within a month before their death.[38,39] Although the US Preventive Services Task Force concluded that evidence was insufficient to support routine screening of adolescents for suicide risk in primary care settings, Gardner and colleagues[40] found that pediatric primary care is a feasible setting in which to screen youths for suicide risk and link them with mental health services. In terms of interventions with potential to rapidly and substantially reduce suicide rates in the United States, Bridge and colleagues[41] prioritized suicide prevention research in 2 areas: (1) increasing access to primary care–based behavioral health interventions for depressed youth and (2) improving continuity of care for youth who present to emergency departments after a suicide attempt.

Zuni American Indian Life Skills Program

The Zuni American Indian Life Skills program involves teaching coping skills tailored to Native American culture and heritage and has been show to increase suicide intervention skills and decrease hopelessness.[42]

TERTIARY PREVENTION
Psychotherapy

A review by Brown and Jager-Hyman,[43] reports that numerous randomized clinical trials have shown that cognitive-behavioral therapy and other psychotherapies are effective in targeting and reducing suicide ideation and attempts.

Cognitive-behavioral therapy is a time-limited, problem-focused treatment that has been implemented in a variety of populations at increased risk for suicide, such as those with depression, personality disorders, anxiety disorders, substance abuse, and schizophrenia. It has also been used for those with suicide ideation and attempts.[44,45] Because most existing studies have only examined the short-term impact of cognitive-behavioral therapy on suicidal thought and behaviors, more emphasis needs to be placed on examining the long-term impact of cognitive-behavioral therapy.[46]

Dialectical behavior therapy (DBT), a form of cognitive–behavioral therapy, is empirically supported as a treatment for suicidal individuals. DBT was developed in the 1980s by Dr Marsha M. Linehan for those with borderline personality disorder. Standard DBT and DBT with skills training have proven to be effective in reducing suicide attempts in adults and adolescents.[47,48]

Pharmacotherapy

The Treatment of Adolescent Suicide Attempters Study reported that adolescents who received combined treatment, including selective serotonin reuptake inhibitors and psychotherapy showed rates of improvement and remission of depression that were similar to rates observed in nonsuicidal, depressed patients who had received similar treatment.[49] Lithium is recommended in the practice parameters for reducing risk of suicide and suicide attempts in patients with bipolar disorder and major depressive disorder.[50] In a systematic review of randomized trials conducted by Cipriani and colleagues,[51] it was found that lithium reduces the risk of suicide in people with mood disorder. The mechanisms mediating the "antisuicidal" effect need more study, but although lithium reduces relapse of mood disorder it also seems to reduce aggression and impulsivity.

Safety Plans

Safety plans are brief clinical interventions used with people at high risk for suicide such as those with prior attempt, recent ideation, and psychiatric disorder. A safety plan is a prioritized written list of coping strategies and sources of support that patients can use during or preceding suicidal crises.[52] Safety plans provide patients with something more than just a referral when the opportunity or circumstance for immediate and longer term care is limited. The steps in developing a safety plan, as outlined by Stanley and Brown[52] are (1) recognizing warning signs that may trigger a suicidal crisis, (2) identifying and using internal coping strategies without needing to contact another person, (3) using contacts with people as a means of distraction from suicidal thoughts and urges, (4) contacting family members or friends who may help to resolve a crisis, (5) contacting mental health professionals or agencies, and (6) reducing the potential for use of lethal means. Patients are instructed first to recognize when they are in crisis (step 1) and then to follow steps 2 through 5 as outlined in the plan.

PRIMARY PREVENTION

Primary prevention targets the general population of children and adolescents before suicidal thoughts or behaviors occur and may include a wide range of interventions, such as skills building programs, educational approaches, campaigns targeting stigma reduction, and policies to increase access to health care or restrict access to lethal means.

Means Restriction

Means restriction has been cited as one of the most impactful suicide prevention interventions.[53] This includes firearm safety, construction of barriers at jumping sites, detoxification of domestic gas, improvements in the use of catalytic converters in motor vehicles, restrictions on pesticides, use of lower toxicity antidepressants, changing packaging of medications to blister packs, and restricting sales of lethal hypnotics (ie, barbiturates). The universal approach with the strongest and most consistent evidence of preventing suicide is means restriction and control.[54–56]

The Good Behavior Game

The Good Behavior Game (GBG) is an evidence-based practice that was developed in the 1960s by Barrish, Saunders, and Wolfe.[57] A trial in Baltimore in 1985 and 1986 was the first effectiveness trial involving randomization and long-term follow-up.[58]

The core elements of the GBG as played in the Baltimore trial are that early in first grade the teacher posts the classroom rules and forms 3 heterogeneous teams by gender and behavior. Rewards are group contingent, meaning that teams are rewarded for each child's prosocial behavior and not rewarded when a child is aggressive or disruptive. The GBG was played 3 times a week for 10 minutes early in the year. The time and frequency were extended over the course of the year. Early in first grade, teams win small concrete rewards; later, rewards become more abstract.

Participants in this trial conducted in 1985 and 1986 included 2311 first-grade students (mean age, 6.3 ± 0.45 years) from Baltimore city schools; 50.2% of participants were male, 65.5% African American, and 52.6% qualified for free or reduced price meals. Retention at ages 19 to 22 was 80% and 67% at age 30. Diagnostic and psychosocial assessments were collected in grades 1 to 8 and ages 19/20, 21/22, and 30. Data were collected from children, teachers, peers, and parents. Public records were gathered on arrests, criminal convictions, and deaths. Participants reported on suicide ideation and attempt at ages 19, 21, and 30.

The study design involved 19 schools in matched sets of 3 to 4 in 5 urban areas in East Baltimore. Schools were assigned randomly within sets to an externally matched control school, reading achievement (ML [master learning]) school, and classroom management (GBG) schools. The GBG was implemented over first and second grades in 2 consecutive cohorts of first graders. The first cohort received 40 hours of training in addition to supportive mentoring and monitoring through the year. The second cohort, which served as the sustainability trial, received no additional training and minimal support.

Wilcox and colleagues[59] reported that first graders assigned to GBG classrooms experienced lower incidence of suicidality through childhood, adolescence, and into young adulthood compared with internal GBG controls. They reported one-half the lifetime rates of suicide ideation and attempts compared with their matched controls. As shown in **Table 1**, the GBG had an impact on reducing the incidence of other behavioral outcomes such drug abuse and dependence, alcohol abuse and dependence, regular smoking, antisocial personality disorder, and violent and criminal behavior. A recent study found that although individuals assigned to the GBG intervention did not receive significantly higher social preference scores, highly aggressive children assigned to the GBG received significantly higher peer preference scores as compared with highly aggressive, disruptive control children.[60] This work points to the social benefits of the GBG. Replication is needed of the impact of the GBG on suicide ideation and attempt.

Youth Aware of Mental Health Program

Youth Aware of Mental Health Program (YAM) is a manualized, universal intervention. It involves role play sessions within interactive workshops as well as a 32-page booklet

Table 1
Young adult outcomes in GBG and standard classrooms

Summary of Previously Published Results	GBG (%)	Standard Program (%)
Drug abuse/dependence disorders		
Males only	19	38
Highly aggressive, disruptive males only	29	83
Alcohol abuse/dependence disorders		
Both genders combined	13	20
Regular Smoking		
Males only	7	17
Highly aggressive, disruptive males only	0	25
Antisocial Personality Disorder		
Both genders combined	17	25
Highly aggressive, disruptive males only	41	86
Juvenile court and/or adult incarceration record for violent and criminal behavior		
Highly aggressive, disruptive males only	34	50
Use of school-based services for problems with behavior, feeling, or drugs and alcohol		
Males only	17	33
Suicide ideation		
Females only	9	19
Males only	11	24
Suicide attempt		
Females only	10	20
Males only	10	18

Abbreviation: GBG, Good Behavior Game.
Adapted from Kellam SG, Mackenzie ACL, Brown CH, et al. The good behavior game and the future of prevention and treatment. Addict Sci Clin Pract 2011;6(1):77.

for pupils, 6 educational posters to be displayed in classrooms, and two 1-hour inter-active lectures about mental health at the beginning and end of the intervention.[19] YAM aims to increase mental health awareness, to increase knowledge about depres-sion and anxiety, and to build skills for coping with adverse events and stress. This program proved to reduce suicide attempts over 1 year in a European trial of 3 inter-ventions.[19] Replication of YAM is needed.

SUMMARY AND FUTURE DIRECTIONS

Many suicide prevention programs are listed on the National Registry of Evidence based Programs and Practices but very few have demonstrated evidence of effective-ness from randomized trials. Nearly all widely used programs aim to identify youth af-ter they have already developed identifiable symptoms or after a suicidal crisis has already started, which is an approach that is unlikely to reduce rates of youth suicide in the general population significantly.

For most youth who die by suicide, there are opportunities for intervention before imminent risk and problems develop.[61] Effective prevention programs have been iden-tified that reduce the occurrence and severity of mental, emotional, and behavioral problems that increase risk for suicidal behavior, many offered through schools[62–64]; however, the impact of these programs on reducing suicidal behaviors is unknown at present because evaluators of these interventions have rarely included suicidal behavior in their outcome measures. Identifying the impact of these programs is un-derway as part of the National Institutes of Health Pathways to Prevention program.

To advance upstream suicide prevention, we also recommend identifying other promising intervention settings and strategies. Social media has been in the spotlight owing to rapidly expanding Internet-networked communication, concerns about cyberbullying, and the tendency of vulnerable youth to seek peers on social media instead of help in person. In 2011, Facebook added a feature to report suicidal con-tent, which has been recently updated to pass information to the National Suicide Pre-vention Lifeline. Owing to social media's wide reach to youth isolated from adults and its ability to provide extensive real-time data, this setting has great potential for suicide prevention. We also recommend suicide prevention approaches that integrate the physical and behavioral health domains.[65]

As pointed out by Brent and Brown,[66] for suicide risk screening or GKT to reduce suicides, detection has to be accurate, students and their parents need to follow through with referrals and the treatment has to be effective. Because a national survey indicates that community treatment for suicidal young people has not established consistent effectiveness,[67] interventions such as the GBG or YAM, which build skills, and Sources of Strength, which builds communication ties to adults, seem to be wise suicide prevention investments. Replication and cost-effectiveness studies of these primary prevention approaches are needed. A greater investment is required to build infrastructure to support financing and sustaining large-scale, coordinated suicide prevention efforts and research.

REFERENCES

1. Web-based Injury Statistics Query and Reporting System (WISQARS) [Online]. National Center for Injury Prevention and Control, Centers for Disease Control and Prevention; 2016. Available at: www.cdc.gov/ncipc/wisqars. Accessed January 7, 2016.

2. National Action Alliance for Suicide Prevention. 2012 national strategy for suicide prevention: goals and objectives for action. Washington, DC: US Department of Health and Human Services; 2012.

3. National Action Alliance for Suicide Prevention: Research Prioritization Task Force. A prioritized research agenda for suicide prevention: an action plan to save lives. Rockville (MD): National Institute of Mental Health and the Research Prioritization Task Force; 2014.

4. Nock MK, Borges G, Bromet EJ, et al. Suicide and suicidal behavior. Epidemiol Rev 2008;30:133–54.

5. O'Carroll PW, Berman AL, Maris RW, et al. Beyond the tower of babel: a nomenclature for suicidology. Suicide Life Threat Behav 1996;26(3):237–52.

6. Silverman MM, Berman AL, Sanddal ND, et al. Rebuilding the tower of Babel: a revised nomenclature for the study of suicide and suicidal behaviors. Part 2: suicide-related ideations, communications, and behaviors. Suicide Life Threat Behav 2007;37(3):264–77.

7. Crosby AE, Ortega L, Melanson C. Self-directed violence surveillance: uniform definitions and recommended data elements, version 1.0. Atlanta (GA): Centers for Disease Control and Prevention, National Center for Injury Prevention and Control; 2011.

8. Shaffer D, Craft L. Methods of adolescent suicide prevention. J Clin Psychiatry 1999;60:70–4.

9. Giedd JN, Blumenthal J, Jeffries NO, et al. Brain development during childhood and adolescence: a longitudinal MRI study. Nat Neurosci 1999;2:861–3.

10. Gogtay N, Giedd JN, Lusk L, et al. Dynamic mapping of human cortical development during childhood through early adulthood. Proc Natl Acad Sci U S A 2004; 101:8174–9.

11. Florentine JB, Crane C. Suicide prevention by limiting access to methods: a review of theory and practice. Soc Sci Med 2010;70:1626–32.

12. Brown CH, Wyman PA, Guo J, et al. Dynamic wait-listed designs for randomized trials: new designs for prevention of youth suicide. Clin Trials 2006;3:259–71.

13. Data and Surveillance Task Force of the National Action Alliance for Suicide Prevention. Improving national data systems for surveillance of suicide-related events. Am J Prev Med 2014;47:S122–9.

14. Walrath C, Garraza LG, Reid H, et al. Impact of the Garrett Lee Smith youth suicide prevention program on suicide mortality. Am J Public Health 2015;105:986–93.

15. Gould MS, Greenberg T, Velting DM, et al. Youth suicide risk and preventive interventions: a review of the past 10 years. J Am Acad Child Adolesc Psychiatry 2003;42:386–405.

16. Burnette C, Ramchand R, Ayer L. Office of the Secretary of Defense. Santa Monica, CA: RAND Corporation; 2015. Available at: http://www.sprc.org/library_resources/items/gatekeeper-training-suicide-prevention-theoretical-model-and-review-empirica. Accessed January 7, 2016.

17. Wyman PA, Brown CH, Inman J, et al. Randomized trial of a gatekeeper program for suicide prevention: 1-year impact on secondary school staff. J Consult Clin Psychol 2008;76(1):104–15.

18. Sareen J, Isaak C, Bolton SL, et al. Gatekeeper training for suicide prevention in first nations community members: a randomized controlled trial. Depress Anxiety 2013;30:1021–9.

19. Wasserman D, Hoven CW, Wasserman C, et al. School-based suicide prevention programmes: the SEYLE cluster-randomised, controlled trial. Lancet 2015;385: 1536–44.

20. LoMurray M. Sources of strength facilitators guide: suicide prevention peer gate-keeper training. Bismarck (ND): The North Dakota Suicide Prevention Project; 2005.
21. Wyman PA, Brown CH, LoMurray M, et al. An outcome evaluation of the Sources of Strength suicide prevention program delivered by adolescent peer leaders in high schools. Am J Public Health 2010;100:1653–61.
22. Bearman PS, Moody J. Suicide and friendships among American adolescents. Am J Public Health 2004;94:89–95.
23. Wyman PA, Petrova M, Schmeelk-Cone K, et al. A method for assessing implementation success of a peer-led suicide prevention program. Implementation Science 2015;10(Suppl 1):A42.
24. Centers for Disease Control and Prevention, National Center for Injury Prevention and Control. Strategic direction for the prevention of suicidal behavior: Promoting individual, family, and community connectedness to prevent suicidal behavior. 2008. Available at: http://www.cdc.gov/violenceprevention/suicide/prevention. html. Accessed January 1, 2016.
25. Asarnow JR, Carlson GA, Guthrie D. Coping strategies, self-perceptions, hopelessness, and perceived family environments in depressed and suicidal children. J Consult Clin Psychol 1987;55:361–6.
26. Rotheram-Borus MJ, Trautman PD, Dopkins SC, et al. Cognitive style and pleasant activities among female adolescent suicide attempters. J Consult Clin Psychol 1990;58:554–61.
27. Rogers EM. Diffusion of innovations. 5th edition. New York: The Free Press; 2003. p. 221.
28. Valente TW. Network models of the diffusion of innovations. Cresskill (NJ): Hampton Press; 1995.
29. Schilling EA, Aseltine RH Jr, James A. The SOS suicide prevention program: further evidence of efficacy and effectiveness. Prev Sci 2015. [Epub ahead of print].
30. Aseltine RH Jr, DeMartino R. An outcome evaluation of the SOS suicide prevention program. Am J Public Health 2004;94:446–51.
31. Aseltine RH Jr, James A, Schilling EA, et al. Evaluating the SOS suicide prevention program: a replication and extension. BMC Public Health 2007;7:161.
32. Schilling EA, Lawless M, Buchanan L, et al. "Signs of Suicide" shows promise as a middle school suicide prevention program. Suicide Life Threat Behav 2014;44: 653–67.
33. Haas A, Koestner B, Rosenberg J, et al. An interactive web-based method of outreach to college students at risk for suicide. J Am Coll Health 2008;57(1):15–22.
34. Spitzer RL, Kroenke K, Williams JBW, et al. Validity and utility of a self-report version of PRIME-MD: the PHQ primary care study. JAMA 1999;282:1737–44.
35. Spitzer RL, Williams JBW, Kroenke K. Validity and utility of the Patient Health Questionnaire in assessment of 3000 obstetric-gynecologic patients: the PRIME-MD Patient Health Questionnaire Obstetrics-Gynecology Study. Am J Obstet Gynecol 2000;183:759–69.
36. Horowitz LM, Bridge JA, Teach SJ, et al. Ask Suicide-Screening Questions (ASQ): a brief instrument for the pediatric emergency department. Arch Pediatr Adolesc Med 2012;166:1170–6.
37. Kruesi MJ, Grossman J, Pennington JM, et al. Suicide and violence prevention: parent education in the emergency department. J Am Acad Child Adolesc Psychiatry 1999;38:250–5.
38. Luoma JB, Martin CE, Pearson JL. Contact with mental health and primary care providers before suicide: a review of the evidence. Am J Psychiatry 2002;159: 909–16.

39. Andersen UA, Andersen M, Rosholm JU, et al. Contacts to the health care system prior to suicide: a comprehensive analysis using registers for general and psychiatric hospital admissions, contacts to general practitioners and practising specialists and drug prescriptions. Acta Psychiatr Scand 2000; 102:126–34.

40. Gardner W, Klima J, Chisolm D, et al. Screening, triage, and referral of patients who report suicidal thought during a primary care visit. Pediatrics 2010;125:945–52.

41. Bridge JA, Horowitz LM, Fontanella CA, et al. Prioritizing research to reduce youth suicide and suicidal behavior. Am J Prev Med 2014;47:S229–34.

42. Lafromboise TD, Lewis HA. The Zuni life skills development program: a school/community-based suicide prevention intervention. Suicide Life Threat Behav 2008;38(3):343–53.

43. Brown GK, Jager-Hyman S. Evidence-based psychotherapies for suicide prevention: future directions. Am J Prev Med 2014;47:S186–94.

44. Slee N, Garnefski N, van der Leeden R, et al. Cognitive–behavioural intervention for self-harm: randomised controlled trial. Br J Psychiatry 2008;192:202–11.

45. Stanley B, Brown G, Brent DA, et al. Cognitive-behavioral therapy for suicide prevention (CBT-SP): treatment model, feasibility, and acceptability. J Am Acad Child Adolesc Psychiatry 2009;48:1005–13.

46. Thoma N, Pilecki B, McKay D. Contemporary cognitive behavior therapy: a review of theory, history, and evidence. Psychodyn Psychiatry 2015;43:423–62.

47. Linehan MM, Korslund KE, Harned MS, et al. Dialectical behavior therapy for high suicide risk in individuals with borderline personality disorder: a randomized clinical trial and component analysis. JAMA Psychiatry 2015;72:475–82.

48. Katz LY, Cox BJ, Gunasekara S, et al. Feasibility of dialectical behavior therapy for suicidal adolescent inpatients. Child Adolesc Psychiatry 2004;43:276–82.

49. Vitiello B, Brent DA, Greenhill LL, et al. Depressive symptoms and clinical status during the Treatment of Adolescent Suicide Attempters (TASA) Study. J Am Acad Child Adolesc Psychiatry 2009;48:997–1004.

50. Jacobs DG, Baldessarini RJ, Conwell Y, et al. Practice guideline for the assessment and treatment of patients with suicidal behaviors. Arlington, VA: American Psychiatric Association; 2010.

51. Cipriani A, Hawton K, Stockton S, et al. Lithium in the prevention of suicide in mood disorders: updated systematic review and meta-analysis. BMJ 2013;346: f3646.

52. Stanley B, Brown GK. Safety planning intervention: a brief intervention to Mitigate suicide risk. Cogn Behav Pract 2012;19:256–64.

53. Mann JJ, Apter A, Bertolote J, et al. Suicide prevention strategies: a systematic review. JAMA 2005;294:2064–74.

54. Crifasi CK, Meyers JS, Vernick JS, et al. Effects of changes in permit-to-purchase handgun laws in Connecticut and Missouri on suicide rates. Prev Med 2015;79: 43–9.

55. Anestis MD, Anestis JC. Suicide rates and state laws regulating access and exposure to handguns. Am J Public Health 2015;105:2049–58.

56. Fleegler EW, Lee LK, Monuteaux MC, et al. Firearm legislation and firearm-related fatalities in the United States. JAMA Intern Med 2013;173(9):732–40.

57. Barrish HH, Saunders M, Wolfe MD. Good behavior game: effects of individual contingencies for group consequences and disruptive behavior in a classroom. J Appl Behav Anal 1969;2:119–24.

58. Kellam SG, Brown CH, Poduska JM, et al. Effects of a universal classroom behavior management program in first and second grades on young adult

behavioral, psychiatric, and social outcomes. Drug Alcohol Depend 2008;95: S5–28.

59. Wilcox HC, Kellam SG, Brown CH, et al. The impact of two universal randomized first- and second-grade classroom interventions on young adult suicide ideation and attempts. Drug Alcohol Depend 2008;95:S60–73.

60. Newcomer AR, Roth KB, Kellam SG, et al. Higher childhood peer reports of social preference mediates the impact of the good behavior game on suicide attempt. Prev Sci 2015. [Epub ahead of print].

61. Wyman PA. Developmental approach to prevent adolescent suicides: research pathways to effective upstream preventive interventions. Am J Prev Med 2014; 47:S251–6.

62. Botvin GJ, Griffin KW, Diaz T, et al. Preventing illicit drug use in adolescents: long-term follow-up data from a randomized control trial of a school population. Addict Behav 2000;25:769–74.

63. Hawkins JD, Oesterle S, Brown EC, et al. Results of a type 2 translational research trial to prevent adolescent drug use and delinquency: a test of communities that care. Arch Pediatr Adolesc Med 2009;163:789–98.

64. Spoth RL, Redmond C, Shin C. Randomized trial of brief family interventions for general populations: adolescent substance use outcomes 4 years following baseline. J Consult Clin Psychol 2001;69:627–42.

65. Sibold J, Edwards E, Murray-Close D, et al. Physical activity, sadness, and suicidality in bullied US adolescents. J Am Acad Child Adolesc Psychiatry 2015; 54(10):808–15.

66. Brent DA, Brown CH. Effectiveness of school-based suicide prevention programmes. Lancet 2015;385:1489–91.

67. Nock MK, Green JG, Hwang I, et al. Prevalence, correlates, and treatment of lifetime suicidal behavior among adolescents: results from the National Comorbidity Survey Replication Adolescent Supplement. JAMA Psychiatry 2013;70:300–10.

Bullying

David C. Rettew, MD[a],*, Sara Pawlowski, MD[b]

KEYWORDS

- Bullying • Prevention • Olweus • Peer aggression

KEY POINTS

- Bullying refers to repetitive and intentional peer aggression where there exists a power imbalance.
- Research has increasingly documented the serious and long-term behavioral and health consequences of bullying.
- Several strategies have demonstrated efficacy in addressing and preventing bullying on the individual level and more broadly within schools and communities.

INTRODUCTION

Bullying is a complex and widespread public health issue that affects children of all ages and adults. For decades, the experience of being bullied as a child has been viewed as an unpleasant but generally harmless rite of passage that carries with it few long-term consequences. Portrayals of bullying in countless books and movies depict bully victims as inevitably resilient and victorious, whereas the bully eventually meets with justice. In the real world, however, such an optimistic view has been tempered by some high-profile suicides coupled with an accumulating literature that has revealed, to the surprise of many, how serious and widespread the sequelae of bullying can be. Current thinking now reflects an understanding of bullying as a social and cultural phenomenon associated with long-term serious physical and psychological consequences for bullies, victims, and those who oscillate between both roles (bully-victims). With this increased concern about bullying has fortunately come a surge of research directed at advancing basic understanding of bullying behavior and at guiding antibullying interventions on the individual and community level. The following sections address several features of bullying including epidemiology,

Financial Disclosure: Dr D.C. Rettew reports royalties from W.W. Norton & Company and Psychology Today. Dr S. Pawlowski reports no financial relationships with commercial interests.
[a] Child & Adolescent Psychiatry Fellowship, Pediatric Psychiatry Clinic, University of Vermont College of Medicine, 1 South Prospect Street, Arnold 3, Burlington, VT 05401, USA; [b] Child & Adolescent Psychiatry, University of Vermont Medical Center, 1 South Prospect Street, Arnold 3, Burlington, VT 05401, USA
* Corresponding author. 1 South Prospect Street, Arnold 3, Burlington, VT 05401.
E-mail address: david.rettew@med.uvm.edu

Child Adolesc Psychiatric Clin N Am 25 (2016) 235–242
http://dx.doi.org/10.1016/j.chc.2015.12.002   childpsych.theclinics.com
1056-4993/16/$ – see front matter © 2016 Elsevier Inc. All rights reserved.

psychological and physical impact, and the role of health care providers in bullying detection, intervention, and prevention.

DEFINITION AND PHENOMENOLOGY OF BULLYING

Bullying is often defined as repetitive and intentional aggressive behavior by one individual or group against another in situations where there exists some sort of power differential between the bully and the victim in terms of physical size, social status, or other features.[1] Bullying behavior can include anything from name-calling to outright physical assault. What has been termed relational bullying can involve such actions as spreading rumors or the active ignoring or exclusion of certain individuals. Bullying can also occur online in the form of text messages, emails, and social media posts.

At least moderate levels of bullying are estimated to occur in about 30% of school-age children, although estimates vary widely because of differences in definition and methodology.[2] One piece of good news, however, is that there is evidence that the prevalence of bullying in the United States may be decreasing.[3] A recent report from the Department of Education cites a rate of bullying at school of 22%, the lowest level since the data were gathered in 2005 (http://nces.ed.gov/blogs/nces/post/measuring-student-safety-bullying-rates-at-school).

School grounds remain the most common site for bullying, and physical appearance is the most common target of bullying behavior.[4] Sexual orientation is also a common focus. Boys tend to bully more than girls, although this difference is diminished, if not reversed, when the definition includes more relational types of bullying.[5] Furthermore, boys tend to be more likely to bully those outside of their core group of friends, whereas girls are more likely to bully individuals within their social network.

Longitudinal studies reveal some trends regarding bullying through childhood and adolescence. Early bullying can be readily identified in elementary school children but tends to peak in the middle school years and early adolescence. It often diminishes later in adolescence and adulthood, although there remains a minority of youth who increase their level of bullying through adolescence.[6]

Many studies of bullying have traditionally divided groups of children into those who are (1) bullies only, (2) victims only, and those who are (3) both bullies and victims. Other groups that are occasionally identified are bystanders, defenders, assistors, and reinforcers.[7] Although broad terms, such as bullies, are admittedly overly heterogeneous,[8] efforts have been slow to identify potentially more meaningful subtypes and categories. For example, there may be a group of more "alpha" bullies who tend to be popular, more socially dominant, and with less comorbid psychopathology in contrast to another group of bullies who are more dysregulated ("delta" bullies), less socially skilled, and with more associated behavioral problems. Such distinctions could prove meaningful with regard to future research studies and intervention strategies.

NEGATIVE EFFECTS OF BULLYING

The negative effects of bullying are being increasingly appreciated. Indeed, the magnitude of these effects has surprised mental health professionals and the general public. Bullying is estimated to cause children to miss approximately 160,000 days of school each year according to the National Education Association (http://www.ncpc.org/topics/bullying/what-parents-can-do). A loss of up to 1.5 letter grades because of bullying has also been documented during the middle school years.[9] In the area of mental health and psychiatric disorders, bullying has been linked to future levels of anxiety, depression, suicidality, psychosis, and self-harm behaviors, among others.[10–12]

Overall, the level of trauma with regard to bullying has been found to be roughly equivalent to a child being placed outside of the home[13] and may be more severe than other forms of child maltreatment.[14] Outside of direct psychiatric illness, bullying in childhood has also been associated with higher levels of chronic inflammation in adulthood.[15]

For bullies, themselves, the picture is more mixed. Some studies have demonstrated that many bullies, especially those who also have been bully victims, show elevated levels of psychopathology. Other studies, however, show evidence that more "pure" bullies may have lower rates of mental health problems.[16]

BULLYING DETECTION AND INTERVENTION

Many organizations including the American Academy of Pediatrics and the American Academy of Child and Adolescent Psychiatry have emphasized the role of mental health professionals and other health care providers in reducing and preventing bullying. Giving anticipatory guidance, using effective tools to screen for bullying, and making efforts in early intervention can lead to marked differences in the lives of many children and their families. In these ways, primary care and mental health professionals can be in the forefront of prevention of this social epidemic.

This section discusses bullying identification and then presents an overview of prevention strategies, at the clinical practice level and in the larger community context, to outline possible avenues for advocacy that can occur in a range of settings. A useful resource for clinicians is the Connected Kids Web site from the American Academy of Pediatrics (www.aap.org), which provides information about screening, family guidance, and bullying interventions with a focus on violence prevention in routine health care visits.

Identification

A first step in preventing bullying is effective screening in response to signs of bullying and victimization. Interventions against bullying start with early detection, as shown in **Box 1**. Often bullying is subtle and hidden, especially with regard to more covert relational bullying. It is also important to keep in mind that children tend to err on the side of underreporting because of the fear of repercussions or feelings of disempowerment and shame.

When bullying victims do present for help, it is often in the context of general somatic complaints without an obvious cause. Victims may also show symptoms of social phobia, depression, or attention problems. They may also experience poorer grades, or begin missing school.[17] Many of these symptoms parallel those seen in victims of domestic violence.

Box 1
Opportunities for bullying prevention in pediatric primary care (middle childhood)

1. Screen for bullying risk factors including sudden reports of changes in behavior (more depressed, suicidal ideation), truancy, and chronic somatic symptoms without a discernable cause.

2. Provide anticipatory guidance for elementary school students especially those at risk (perceived as anxious, weaker than other children) before the peak bullying age in middle school.

3. Discuss openly, directly, and gently a child's experience at school. Do not dispute a child's report of bullying even if it is not perceived by parents or teachers.

4. Advocate for schools to adopt elements of effective bullying prevention programs.

If bullying is suspected, further questions are warranted. These may include inquiries found in **Box 2**. Such questions can open the topic and reveal possible avenues for intervention, such as a more focused pediatric psychiatric referral or a discussion with the school principal to advocate for effective school-based interventions. For some children who seem reluctant to discuss their own personal history about bullying, initial questions that refer to the general climate of the school (eg, "Is bullying a problem at your school?") can sometimes help begin a conversation. It may also be worthwhile to remind young patients about the protection and limits of confidential discussions.

Individual Level Interventions

Bully victims

Once bullying is suspected or uncovered, there are some general principles that can guide individual level interventions in the office. Clinicians may find it helpful to differentiate lower levels of bullying (name calling, teasing) from higher levels (overt threats, physical violence, and intimidation), keeping in mind that all forms can be potentially harmful.

For lower-level bullying, the following points are helpful to remember when working with kids directly and in helping parents help their children:

- Do not underestimate the power of sympathetic listening. Overt expressions to a child that he or she does not deserve this and that such behaviors are really hurtful can be very important to many kids. Positive experiences with friends and families can also go a long way to counteract a negative encounter with a bully.
- Coach bully victims about how to respond. The old adage of telling a bully that he or she is hurting your feelings has been replaced with advice to react emotionally as little as possible. Some children also are helped by rehearsing specific responses or learning to join nonthreatening peer groups during higher risk activities.
- If the bullying is occurring online, encourage kids to save the texts or social media posts if needed as evidence.
- Consider the option of an anonymous report to a school principal or guidance counselor. As an example, although school personnel may be unable to make a direct response, they might be able to provide more monitoring at high-risk areas, such as bathrooms, school buses, or locker rooms.

Box 2
Sample bullying screening questions

- I'd like to hear about how school is going. How many good friends do you have in school? (Child) Is your child being picked on at school? (Parent)
- Do you ever feel afraid to go to school? Why?
- Do other kids ever bully you at school, in your neighborhood or online? Who bullies you? When and where does it happen? What do they say or do?
- What do you do if you see other kids being bullied?
- Who can you go to for help if you or someone you know is being bullied?
- When you go for help, what is done about it?

Data from US Department of Health & Human Services. How to talk about bullying. Available at: www.stopbullying.gov. Accessed August 7, 2015.

For higher levels of bullying, the role of the school, parents, and sometimes even law enforcement is more prominent. The government Web site www.stopbullying.gov includes several helpful suggestions and guidelines. Although the response to help the victim is often similar here as with lower-level bullying, more emphasis is placed on adults to determine more precisely what has happened and to design a response for the bully, if indicated. Many states now have mandatory bullying prevention and intervention policies. Although parents of bullying victims may have strong and natural urges to confront directly the parents of the alleged bully, this step often does not help the situation and can often makes things worse. Finally, if there is evidence that bullying is having a strong negative impact on the child, a more in-depth evaluation to rule out anxiety disorders, depression, and the presence of any suicidal or homicidal thinking should be strongly considered.

Bullies

There is less information on how to identify bullies and how to intervene with bullies individually. Keeping in mind that many youth who bully themselves have histories of victimization and comorbid psychopathology, some may benefit from further evaluation and treatment. Alerting parents to bullying behavior and offering parent behavioral guidance can also be useful, although it should not be assumed that bullies necessarily come from dysfunctional households. According to stopbullying.gov, some interventions that are not particularly effective include group therapy, "zero tolerance" approaches involving suspension or expulsion, or mediation sessions between the victim and bully.

School- and Community-Based Programs

With the increased awareness of the consequences of bullying have come many comprehensive strategies for prevention and intervention that target bullies, victims, bystanders, teachers, educators, community members, families, and health care practitioners. In the context of bullying as a social phenomenon, many efforts are directed at attempting to change cultural attitudes, with strategies that target the social climate of schools and the greater community.

One of the pioneers in bullying research is Dan Olweus, a researcher on this topic since the 1970s at the University of Bergen in Norway. His work was inspired by several tragic adolescent deaths by suicide that were linked to bullying. The Olweus Bullying Prevention Program is arguably the most researched and widely adopted bullying prevention program in the world.[1] Its aim is to create a supportive school climate through repeated surveys of the school climate from staff, parents, and students. The program recommends the use of varied interventions that include group meetings and interactive videos to foster this change in climate over time.

The degree to which various antibullying programs have been scrutinized and tested varies considerably. The literature on bullying intervention has only recently expanded to allow for a more systematic synthesis of findings across studies. In a 2008 meta-analysis by Merrell and coworkers[18] of school bullying intervention research from 1980 through 2004, the authors reviewed whole-school programs versus small group programs or other smaller scale interventions (which often include lessons about bullying, videos, role-playing, and so forth). Most programs demonstrated no significant change in direct bullying behaviors but they often did improve knowledge, attitudes, and self-perceptions about bullying.

Meta-analyses of bullying prevention programs were also performed by Ttofi and Farrington.[19,20] Overall, the authors could not recommend one program but did find some common features of programs that are effective in reducing bullying and victimization. These included the following three elements: (1) presence of parent and teacher training, (2) strict classroom rules for handling bullying, and (3) the implementation of a whole-school antibullying policy. The authors also noted that bullying occurs less often in schools where staff have a shared understanding of what bullying is, have the ability to communicate well with students about unacceptable behavior, intervene nonaggressively but effectively, adopt routines for documenting and following up cases and incidents, and have open and frequent contact with parents.

The KiVa program is an up-and-coming Finnish initiative that claims not only to prevent bullying but to have a strategic plan for when bullying cases arise.[21] What is unique about this program is the admission that bullying will not be completely eradicated with prevention efforts and that there must be systems in place for victims, bullies, and bystanders to address bullying when it occurs. In this way, the KiVa program mirrors substance abuse programs where there must be constant vigilance even after the initial prevention for risk of relapse and an acknowledgment that relapse into a culture of bullying can occur at any time.

CURRENT CONTROVERSIES AND SUMMARY

Although consensus continues to move forward regarding issues related to bullying and bullying intervention, there remain several areas that are controversial and debated. Even the definition of bullying is under scrutiny. The Global Health Initiative for the Prevention of Bullying (http://www.ghipb.org/definition-of-bullying.html), for example, disputes the requirement for intentionality and would include, under bullying, aggressive acts that are the results of a person being impulsive or dysregulated. The conceptualization of a bully is also under debate with some emphasizing bullies as symptomatic individuals who themselves are suffering from mental health problems, whereas others stressing bullies as more socially dominant individuals invoking a strategy to maintain their rank in their peer community. Further research is needed to examine potentially meaningful subtypes when it comes to bullies and bully victims.

With regard to intervention, the provision of schools and communities across the United States and Canada in adopting "zero tolerance" policies with regard to bullying is under scrutiny given the lack of evidence that such interventions are effective. Such strategies stand in contrast to many used in Europe and Australia where policymakers have viewed bullying as a broader social and public health problem requiring comprehensive strategies of prevention. Similarly, the degree to which the bully and victim should directly meet to work out their problems with the help of an adult or even peer mediator is also controversial. Although such mediation sessions are a core component of some programs, some experts find this step ineffective and potentially traumatic for the victim, similar to situations of domestic violence.[22]

It is clear from the research that there is no quick and easy solution to bullying. Clinicians of all types can reduce trauma and help patients and families on the individual level while advocating for effective programs for the broader community. Research suggests that many of the most successful programs induce long-term shifts in the school culture that can only occur with participation from students, staff, parents, community members, and families. Nevertheless, there remains much to learn on many levels about bullying and the ways that this important public health issue can be more fully addressed and prevented.

REFERENCES

1. Olweus D. Bullying at school: what it is and what we can do. Cambridge (United Kingdom): Blackwell; 1993.

2. Nansel TR, Overpeck M, Pilla RS, et al. Bullying behaviors among US youth: prevalence and association with psychosocial adjustment. JAMA 2001;285(16): 2094–100.

3. Finkolhor D, Turner HA, Shattuck A, et al. Prevalence of childhood exposure to violence, crime, and abuse: results from the national survey of children's exposure to violence. JAMA Pediatr 2015;169(8):746–54.

4. Davis S, Nixon CL. Youth voice project: student insights into bullying and peer mistreatment. Champaign (IL): Research Press Publishers; 2015.

5. Coyne SM, Archer J, Elsea M. "We're not friends anymore unless…": the frequency and harmfulness of indirect, relational, and social aggression. Aggress Behav 2006;32:294–307.

6. Pepler D, Jiang D, Craig W, et al. Developmental trajectories of bullying and associated factors. Child Dev 2008;79(2):325–38.

7. Huitsing G, Veenstra R. Bullying in classrooms: participant roles from a social network perspective. Aggress Behav 2012;38(6):494–509.

8. Vaillancourt T, Hymel S, McDougall P. Bullying is power: implications for school-based intervention strategies. J Appl Sch Psychol 2003;19:157–76.

9. Juvonen J, Wang Y, Espinoza G. Bullying experiences and compromised academic performance across middle school grades. J Early Adolesc 2011; 31(1):152–73.

10. Arseneault L, Bowes L, Shakoor S. Bullying victimization in youths and mental health problems: 'much ado about nothing'? Psychol Med 2010;40(5): 717–29.

11. Arseneault L, Walsh E, Trzesniewski K, et al. Bullying victimization uniquely contributes to adjustment problems in young children: a nationally representative cohort study. Pediatrics 2006;118(1):130–8.

12. Wolke D, Copeland WE, Angold A, et al. Impact of bullying in childhood on adult health, wealth, crime, and social outcomes. Psychol Sci 2013;24(10):1958–70.

13. Takizawa R, Maughan B, Arseneault L. Adult health outcomes of childhood bullying victimization: evidence from a five-decade longitudinal British birth cohort. Am J Psychiatry 2014;171(7):777–84.

14. Copeland WE, Wolke D, Angold A, et al. Adult psychiatric outcomes of bullying and being bullied by peers in childhood and adolescence. JAMA Psychiatry 2013;70(4):419–26.

15. Copeland WE, Wolke D, Lereya ST, et al. Childhood bullying involvement predicts low-grade systemic inflammation into adulthood. Proc Natl Acad Sci U S A 2014; 111(21):7570–5.

16. Koh JB, Wong JS. Survival of the fittest and the sexiest: evolutionary origins of adolescent bullying. J Interpers Violence 2015. [Epub ahead of print].

17. Zimmerman FJ, Glew GM, Christakis DA, et al. Early cognitive stimulation, emotional support, and television watching as predictors of subsequent bullying among grade-school children. Arch Pediatr Adolesc Med 2005;159(4): 384–8.

18. Merrell KW, Gueldner BA, Ross SW, et al. How effective are school bullying intervention programs? A meta-analysis of intervention research. Sch Psychol Q 2008; 23(1):26–42.

19. Ttofi MM, Farrington DP. Effectiveness of school-based programs to reduce bullying: a systematic and meta-analytic review. J Exp Criminol 2011;7:27–56.

20. Ttofi MM, Farrington DP, Baldry CA. Effectiveness of programs to reduce school bullying: a systematic review. Stockholm (Sweden): Swedish National Council for Crime Prevention; 2008.

21. Karna A, Voeten M, Little TD, et al. Going to scale: a nonrandomized nationwide trial of the KiVa antibullying program for grades 1-9. J Consult Clin Psychol 2011; 79(6):796–805.
22. Cohen R. Stop mediating these conflicts now! The school mediator: peer mediation insights from the desk of Richard Cohen. Watertown, MA: School Mediation Associates electronic newsletter; 2002. Available at: www. schoolmediation.com. Accessed August 7, 2015.

Prevention of Youth Violence

A Public Health Approach

Aradhana Bela Sood, MD, MSHA[a,b,]*, Steven J. Berkowitz, MD[c]

KEYWORDS

- Youth violence • Violence prevention • Public health and violence

KEY POINTS

- Youth violence is a major public health issue in the United States.
- The relationship between child maltreatment, family dysfunction, and youth violence is well established.
- A public health approach to youth violence prevention should be a long-term strategic plan for communities.

INTRODUCTION

Although youth violence appears to have declined over the past 20 years, the perpetration of violence by youth continues to be a major issue in the nation impacting all aspects of society. Violence remains a leading cause of morbidity and mortality in youth.

This review first discusses the national statistics regarding youth violence, identifies some of its known causes, explores violence prevention in children and youth from a public health perspective, focuses on models and interventions that (1) explicitly target youth violence and (2) have been shown to be effective by high-quality research with a primary focus on perpetration of violence against others. The article discusses the role of child and adolescent mental health practitioners as advocates for prevention both in program implementation and legislation. Although the enumeration of program exemplars is not exhaustive, each of the ones included have evidence to impact violence prevention and contain elements complementary to each other.

[a] Department of Psychiatry, Virginia Commonwealth University, 515 North 10th Street, Richmond, VA 23298, USA; [b] Department of Pediatrics, Virginia Commonwealth University, 515 N 10th Street, Richmond, VA 23298, USA; [c] Department of Psychiatry, Perelman School of Medicine, University of Pennsylvania, Hall Mercer Building, 245 South 8th Street, Philadelphia, PA 19107, USA
* Corresponding author.
E-mail address: Bela.sood@vcuhealth.org

Child Adolesc Psychiatric Clin N Am 25 (2016) 243–256
http://dx.doi.org/10.1016/j.chc.2015.11.004
1056-4993/16/$ – see front matter © 2016 Elsevier Inc. All rights reserved.

SCOPE OF THE PROBLEM

A 2010 report from the Centers for Disease Control and Prevention (CDC) stated that youth homicide was the second leading cause of death among people ages 15 to 24 years and the fourth leading cause of death among youth ages 10 to 14 years.[1] This rate has been consistent over the past several years and also underscores the disparity among homicide victims. Of those 10 to 24 years old, 86% were male and homicide was the leading cause of death for African American individuals; the second leading cause of death for Hispanic individuals; and the third leading cause of death for American Indian and Alaska Native individuals.[1]

In 2011, the CDC reported that 707,212 young people ages 10 to 24 were treated in emergency departments for injuries sustained from physical assaults.[2] In a 2011 survey of a nationally representative sample of high school students, 3.9% reported being in a physical fight at least once in the previous year that caused injuries that had to be treated by a doctor or nurse.[3] In the same 2011 survey, 32.8% reported being in a physical fight in the previous year: males (40.7%) and females (24.4%); 16.6% reported carrying a weapon (gun, knife, or club) on one or more days in the 30 days preceding the survey (males, 25.9%, and females, 6.8%), with 5.1% carrying a gun (males 8.6%, and females, 1.4%).[4] Last, close to 800,000 youth ages 10 to 24 years were treated in emergency departments for nonfatal violence-related injuries in 2013.[5]

School violence is also a major issue, and bullying appears to be on the rise. According to the same 2011 survey, (1) 20.1% of students reported being bullied on school property, (2) 16.2% reported being bullied, (3) 12% reported being in a physical fight on school property, (4) 5.9% did not go to school on 1 or more days in the previous 30 days because they felt unsafe, and (5) 7.4% reported being threatened or injured with a weapon on school property at least once in the year preceding the survey.[5]

The economic burden of youth violence represents another cause for distress. Each year, youth homicides and assault-related injuries result in an estimated $16 billion in combined medical and work loss costs.[2] These statistics are a likely underestimate of actual youth violence and do not address the physical and emotional toll that these experiences take on youth, their families, and their communities.

CAUSES AND CORRELATIONS

Violence is not just limited to individuals, and can become a public health problem for entire communities. The values, attitudes, and interpersonal skills of adults that children are exposed to significantly impact the acquisition of prosocial or violent behaviors in children.[6] The influence of parents, family members, and important adults shape the beliefs of the child in a significant manner; however, the influence of school and the neighborhood also plays an important role in attitudes and behaviors of children toward violence. A focus on one or the other factor can only produce marginal impact on desired outcomes.[7]

The causes of youth violence are multifactorial and include biological, individual, familial, social, and economic factors. Risk factors for violence could be due to individual characteristics in the child, such as social and cognitive deficits, or could be driven by familial factors, such as an early exposure to violence, alcohol abuse in parents, parental divorce, domestic violence, lack of supervision with negative adult or peer influences that espouse a culture of violence, or factors in the community, such as violence in schools that have a coercive social climate and condone bullying, intimidation, and a lack of support for prosocial behavior.[8,9] Most studies point to the finding that the most preventable causal relationship to youth violence is exposure to violence and maltreatment in the home.[10–12] Multiple studies have documented that children's and adolescent's exposure to familial violence, dysfunction, and victimization predicts violent behavior.[13–15]

In the individual child, early warning signs of violence[16] can take the form of social withdrawal and isolation. This is often preceded by actual rejection from peers or family or a subjective feeling of rejection from them. Academic underperformance and gradually eroding self-esteem generates both overt and covert aggression. Creative work reflecting the anger may provide an outlet for expressing the violent feelings. Bullying behavior and intimidation of others and finally identification with a peer group that serves to provide temporary emotional shelter, such as gangs, sets into motion a lifelong propensity for violence. Inappropriate access to and use of firearms, and the use of violence and coercion for conflict resolution all cement violent tendencies in an individual.[17] Such individual factors can become culturally acceptable to an entire community. It is not uncommon for youth in such communities to have a sense of foreshortened future and resulting insensitivity to danger or self-preservation.[18]

Studies have found abused and neglected children to be 25% more likely to become delinquent, experience teen pregnancy, and show low academic achievement.[19] A longitudinal study found that physically abused children were at greater risk of being arrested as juveniles and were less likely to have graduated from high school and more likely to have been a teen parent.[20] A National Institute of Justice study indicated that being abused or neglected as a child increased the likelihood of arrest as a juvenile by 59%. Maltreatment increased the likelihood of adult criminal behavior by 28% and violent crime by 30%.[21] Among offenders, experiencing childhood physical abuse and other forms of maltreatment leads to higher rates of self-reported total offending, violent offending, and property offending, even after controlling for previous delinquent behavior.[21]

Currently, there has been a great deal of interest in the Adverse Childhood Experiences (ACE) study, which demonstrates a graded relationship between 10 adverse childhood experiences in the areas of abuse, neglect, and household dysfunction and a range of negative outcomes in health, behavior, and functioning.[22] One recent study compared the number of ACEs of 64,329 youth who had been involved in the Florida Juvenile Justice system. The juvenile offenders were 13 times less likely to report zero ACEs (2.8% vs 36%) and 4 times more likely to report 4 or more ACEs (50% vs 13%) when compared with the original Kaiser-Permanente sample.[23]

The National Longitudinal Study of Adolescent Health of 9300 youth focused on the relationship between child maltreatment and youth violence perpetration and intimate partner violence (IPV). The victims were more likely to perpetrate youth violence (up to 6.6% for females and 11.9% for males) and young adult IPV (up to 10.4% for females and 17.2% for males).[24]

APPROACHES TO PREVENTING YOUTH VIOLENCE
Reducing Influence of External Factors

The immediate environment of a youth is the family, the neighborhood, and the school (**Box 1**). For a mental health practitioner, the first need is to ensure safety; examples of this may be the removal of a child from abusive parents or who are providing inadequate or dangerously poor supervision or encouraging an adult to leave an abusive partner whose behavior the child may be witnessing.[16] A family may consider leaving a particular neighborhood with rampant community violence or war. A recovering addict may need to move from the surroundings associated with drug use. These interventions may not be economically feasible, but neighborhoods can be made safer by promoting the safe use and safe storage of weapons, enforcing curfews for

---

Box 1
Key primary prevention strategies for violence prevention

- Increase safe, stable, and nurturing relationships between children and their parents and caregivers.
- Enhance social, emotional, and behavioral development, and enhance opportunities for children and youth.
- Promote respectful, nonviolent intimate partner relationships through individual, community, and societal change.
- Promote individual, family, and community connectedness to prevent suicidal behavior.
- Reduce access to lethal means.
- Change cultural norms that support violence.
- Change the social, environmental, and economic characteristics of schools, workplaces, and communities that contribute to violence.

Data from Dahlberg LL, Mercy JA. History of violence as a public health problem. Virtual Mentor 2009;11(2):167–72; and Krug EG, Dahlberg LL, Mercy JA, et al. World report on violence and health. Geneva (Switzerland): World Health Organization; 2002.

---

adolescents, and facilitating constructive activities for youth to engage in after school hours and on weekends.[25–27]

Preventing Violence Using a Public Health Approach

Before selecting evidence-based interventions to address violence, the venue for where the intervention is implemented requires careful thought. A child or youth spends time in the home, school, playgrounds, faith-based programs, day care centers, community centers, and social settings such as malls and movie theaters. For children and adolescents struggling with behavioral issues (high risk) these venues may even be within juvenile detention centers, foster care, and residential and alternative schools programs. These alternative and specialized settings can be either helpful or detrimental to reducing violence, depending on their philosophic approach to programming: trauma informed, strength-based rehabilitative treatment versus coercive/safety-driven treatment philosophy.[28–30]

A collective and holistic public health approach uses the primary, secondary, or tertiary prevention structure to address health problems. All 3 levels of prevention would be essential to address a health issue such as violence in a comprehensive manner. Although it is recognized that community-based universal interventions are expensive, may not reach the targeted population,[6] and pose a challenge for traditional scientific enquiry in that it does not give significant weight to studying the effect of a single intervention, nevertheless a holistic approach has the highest likelihood to produce collective impact on community health.[7] Perhaps the reason for the failure of prevention efforts is the narrow focus of interventions on one aspect or another of a public health issue that is producing isolated impact.[7] Ideally, each level of prevention should be considered important and interventions at varying venues and levels of prevention, complementary to each other, should be implemented. A modified Haddon matrix, is a tool to identify factors operating before, during, and after a condition under scrutiny and adds mediating factors that could impede implementation, such as cost, safety, efficacy, equity, stigmatization, and impact of the countermeasures.[31]

Using the public health model, let's take homicide as an example of a high-stakes behavior that incurs significant emotional and economic toll on any community. A public health approach to reduce homicides would entail the following steps[6]: (1) detecting and defining the problem: what is the rate of homicide in teens in a geographic area, what are the demographics of the victims, does the community see this as a problem that must be addressed; (2) finding the causes of the problem: through surveys, observation within the community, and combining this information with state and national data to identify why the high rates of homicides exist locally: for example, gang activity versus substance abuse versus lack of prosocial activities/mentoring, easy access to firearms; (3) testing scientifically known interventions that work to prevent the causes identified in (2) and finally implementing effective intervention/s either at the larger/entire community level (primary: parent training, education of law enforcement, school-based climate reengineering, safe housing, mentoring, prosocial leisure time activities) or those at risk (secondary: reduction of access to firearms in high-risk youth; mental health intervention with parents; support of prosocial behaviors in high-risk youth, supervision and mentoring of high-risk youth) or those who are already victims of violence (tertiary: support, counseling, vocational, or other skill set training of gunshot wound victims, reduction of circumstances that have encouraged affiliation with gangs, substance abuse treatment).

EFFECTIVE YOUTH VIOLENCE PREVENTION PROGRAMS
Child, Parent, and Family Program Examples (Primary Prevention)

Nurse-family partnership
Nurse-Family Partnership[32] has nurses visiting the home of pregnant women who are deemed to be at high risk for infant health and developmental problems. Although the focus is initially on the pregnant women, the ultimate goal is to improve parenting and child developmental outcomes. During pregnancy, the nurse visits the home weekly and continues to visit for approximately 2 years after the child is born. A protocol is followed during the visits that involves (1) parent education about how to achieve optimal development for the child during pregnancy and after, (2) gaining support for the mother both during and after pregnancy, and (3) linking the family with health and other needed services.[32]

In a 19-year follow-up of the original Elmira, NY, study, adolescents whose mothers received visits were 60% less likely to have run away, 55% less likely to have been arrested, and 80% less likely to have been convicted of a crime than the control group.[33]

Parent management training–Oregon model
The Parent Management Training–Oregon Model (PMTO)[34] is similar to many parent-training models; however, it is the only model that has been shown to reduce later youth violence. It teaches effective family management skills with the goal of decreasing disruptive and antisocial behaviors in children and youth. PMTO has worked with youth from the ages of 3 to 16 years who have diagnosable disorders as well as delinquent youth and caregivers' maltreatment. PMTO is offered both in multifamily groups and with individual families and can be delivered in almost any setting. Sessions are offered weekly and length of involvement is based on the family's needs and interest; however, the multifamily format is time-limited.[34]

PMTO uses well-established teaching and coaching methods to improve parenting skills. Parents are taught and practice skills such as positive reinforcement by using developmentally appropriate behavioral goals, praising positive behavior, and reward-based behavior charts. Limit setting again uses developmentally appropriate rule setting with reasonable consequences. PMTO places a large emphasis on monitoring and supervision by ensuring that caregivers know their child's whereabouts and receive regular and consistent child care when needed. Parents are coached to have positive and consistent participation with their children by spending "quality time." Last, there is a focus on problem solving, which involves appropriate communication and how to deal fairly with disagreements among family members.[34]

There are several shorter-term follow-up studies of PMTO demonstrating decreases in aggressive and problem behaviors among children whose families participated in PMTO.[34–36] In addition, in a 9-year follow-up of youth of single divorced parents, PMTO demonstrated reduced teacher-reported delinquency and police arrests for boys. For those youth who were arrested, there was a significant delay from time of receiving PMTO to arrest compared with the control condition.[37]

Mentoring programs as a strategy to reduce violence

Mentoring,[38] along with providing opportunities for community service and the development of leadership skills, are additional ways to introduce positive modeling and enhance self-esteem.[26,39] The presence of a positive adult role model to supervise and guide a child's behavior is a key protective factor against violence The absence of such role models, such as a parent or other adults, has been linked to sexual promiscuity, aggression, and unstable employment. Conversely, presence of a mentor in a child's life can reduce truancy, reduce violent behavior, and reduce drug use in youth.[40] Community-based programs, such as Big Brothers and Big Sisters, founded in 1904, is one of the oldest such programs and research supports the positive effect of this program on the mentees tendency for violence, substance abuse, school attendance, and academic performance. Site-based mentoring programs are typically within schools (or churches, detention homes, day care) and their advantage is supervised mentoring with oversight and the possibility of group mentoring. Involvement of parents as participants and getting community support for the funding of mentoring programs enhances the success of such programs and in institutionalizing this within a community.[41,42]

Special Population or High-Risk Youth (Secondary Prevention)

Examples of programs for delinquent youth

Multisystemic therapy Multisystemic Therapy (MST)[43] has been used for youth with a number of antisocial issues. Most of the work and research has focused on youth deemed as conduct disordered or delinquent. MST is a community-based and home-based intensive intervention that attends to the known factors that lead to the development of antisocial behavior and violent behavior in youth. It is multisystemic, as MST therapists work in settings that are known to contribute to antisocial behavior, including the family, peers, school, and community. MST was developed as an alternative to placement in juvenile justice facilities with the hypothesis that lasting change must occur in the youth's own ecology. MST works with parents to gain the necessary skills and supports required to address challenging adolescent behaviors and also works directly with the youth to help them manage and problem solve around the issues that arise with their peers, school, and community.[43]

MST therapists are master's level and have a caseload of approximately 6 families. They provide psychotherapeutic services as well as case coordination for additional needs. Treatment lasts up to 6 months and therapists receive weekly supervision. Although MST interventions are tailored to the particular family and youth, there are common areas that are addressed: (1) parental drug use and psychopathology, (2) poor social support and chronic stress, and (3) poor parenting skills. MST focuses on improving parenting, parental monitoring, and communication and problem solving among family members. Peer interventions attempt to decrease the youth's involvement with antisocial peer groups and increase involvement with prosocial peers.

School interventions focus on improving communication between parents and schools and monitoring the youth's school activities and achievement.[43]

Studies of MST have demonstrated significantly decreased rates of delinquency and violent behavior in youth.[44–46] In a 25-year follow-up, the next oldest sibling had significantly fewer arrests and convictions than the control group siblings.[47]

Multidimensional Treatment Foster Care (now called Treatment Foster Care Oregon) Multidimensional Treatment Foster Care (now called Treatment Foster Care Oregon [TFCO])[48] has demonstrated positive outcomes for adolescents with chronic antisocial behavior. It has reduced the number of arrests, violent offenses, and days incarcerated in boys in the juvenile justice system[49] and in girls demonstrated decreases in the number of days incarcerated, arrests, and self-reported antisocial behavior.[50] Families are recruited from the community and are trained and supervised by TFCO clinicians. The family provides interventions and comprehensive supervision at home, in school, and in the community. Caregivers provide consistent limits with appropriate consequences with an emphasis on positive reinforcement. They mentor and sever the youth's relationship with antisocial peers. Youth are incentivized by using a point system that allows them more independence and less supervision as points are accumulated. Youth receive individual and family therapy, and case management. Case managers supervise and support the youth and their foster families with regular phone calls and weekly foster parent group meetings. TFCO emphasizes learning interpersonal skills and positive social activities. TFCO usually lasts for 6 months with aftercare services available as long is necessary.[51]

Functional family therapy Functional Family Therapy (FFT)[52] is a program for youth and their families who have demonstrated antisocial behaviors. It has demonstrated significant decreases in recidivism in several studies, including violent offenses,[52,53] and a recent meta-analysis of 8 studies of FFT reported a mean effect size of –0.32.[54] FFT is a family therapy model as well with frequent phone contact. In addition, it links the youth and family to a range of social and educational services and in some circumstances youth are monitored by para-professionals after the intervention to ensure that gains are sustained. FFT is provided by master's level clinicians with 10 to 12 cases. It is recommended that programs have an FFT team of 3 to 10 clinicians who are supervised by an FFT consultant. It has 4 phases of treatment that build on each other: (1) motivation phase using principles of motivational interviewing therapy; (2) assessment phase, which evaluates the youth, family, and their ecology; (3) changing behavior using a skills-based approach for parents and youth; and (4) consolidation phase, which focuses on the specific issues and concerns of the family.[52]

Social Cognitive Strategies Within Schools to Reduce Violence (All Levels of Prevention)

A systematic review[55] conducted for the CDC's Guide to Community Services (Community Guide) found that institution of universal school-based programs decreases rates of violence among school-age children and youth. All school program intervention strategies (informational, cognitive/affective, and social-skills building) were associated with a reduction in violent behavior. Over all grades combined, the median effect was a 15% relative reduction in violent behavior, with greatest effect seen at the pre-K/K level (32.4% reduction). Program effects were consistent across grade levels and school environments (socioeconomic status, crime rates). School-based programs for the prevention of violence are effective. Effects were larger for programs involving students at higher risk for aggressive behavior. These data support institutions taking a focused approach that emphasizes prosocial behaviors in children and adolescents and explicitly educating them about violence prevention very early on in their schooling.

The establishment of a *safe school environment* requires the involvement of all connected to a school, including school board members, community leaders, law enforcement, and legislators. Identification of risk factors should generate an alert to needed school or community authorities.[56] Open communication about violence in school settings, coping with potential risk factors, and stopping violent behaviors[57] are important to prevent violence. In such an environment, students and teachers feel comfortable enough to share their concerns about troubled students with appropriate personnel.[58–60] Creating a supportive atmosphere by promoting collegial and friendly attitudes; teaching conflict resolution and stress management; and recognition of individuals who seem to be struggling in performance, socially isolated, or displaying other signs of concern should be emphasized.[59,61] Long-term strategies should include measures to (1) develop supports and interventions for at-risk youth, (2) articulating a zero-tolerance policy for peer-on-peer crime, and (3) pursue a combined safety and rehabilitation model to address student misconduct. Helping children learn skills to resolve problems nonviolently by enhancing their social relationships with peers and improving their ability to read behavioral cues can reduce aggression.[62] Children learn these skill sets in multiple settings, such as schools and neighborhoods, and by observing adults, siblings, peers, and cultural icons. The use of didactic teaching, modeling of prosocial behavior, and positive social interactions in role plays becomes the basis of primary and secondary interventions to emphasize nonviolent behavior in young people.[63] School and community centers are the venues in which these programs can reach a large number of children and youth (universal or primary prevention).

Recognizing the presence of risk factors (both internal and external) and providing treatment for them as early as possible is the ideal.[64,65] The first hurdle that must be overcome is teaching the various school personnel about violence prevention.[66] The prevention of, as well as response to, a violent event requires a multidisciplinary team, including health care providers, educators, social services, lawmakers, and community leaders.[66,67]

School-Based Programs to Reduce Violence

Examples

Promoting alternative thinking strategies Promoting Alternative Thinking Strategies (PATHS)[68] is directed at improving emotional and social capabilities and reducing aggression and behavior problems, as well as improving academics for children in grades K–6. In multiple studies, it has demonstrated a reduction in aggressive and antisocial behaviors.[69–71] PATHS is a universal prevention model used by teachers and counselors. Parental involvement is fostered through letters about school activities and assignments performed with parents at home. PATHS uses a developmentally appropriate grade-by-grade curriculum. PATHS curricula focus on improving cognitive and emotional responses to commonly encountered situations. It is taught in the classroom 2 to 3 times weekly with daily group activities to reinforce lessons. Each lesson has proscribed objectives and a script to ensure fidelity with built-in flexibility based on the classroom's characteristics. Each lesson group builds on the next and focuses on (1) affect recognition, (2) self-esteem, (3) friendships, (4) self-control, and (5) problem solving.[68]

Life Skills Training (LST)[72] is a 3-year universal prevention program of substance abuse and violence for middle schools. LST has shown significant decreases in long-term follow-up of substance use among participants,[72–74] and in one study demonstrated a reduction of 32% in antisocial behavior and a 26% reduction in fighting in the past year at a 3-month follow-up.[75] LST trains students in self-management, social skills, and combating peer pressure. It contains 15 central sessions in the first year, 10 booster sessions in the second year, and 5 boosters in the third year. Teachers use standard pedagogic methods to teach the LSI skills and boosters reinforce the material covered in the first year and emphasize new issues that are confronted as they enter adolescence.[72]

The Olweus bullying prevention program The Olweus Bullying Prevention Program[76] is the most evaluated of antibullying models. Developed in Norway, studies have been replicated in the United States with generally positive results.[77–79] It aims to address bullying at the individual, classroom, and school levels. At the individual level, it works directly with bullies, victims, and their parents. At the classroom level, teachers provide clear, regular, and consistent rules and consequences for bullying and regular class discussion about the rules and the impact of bullying on both the victims and perpetrators. At the school level, students answer a questionnaire about bullying at their school. In the subsequent year, there is a full-day conference in which the program's staff review the findings with school staff and learn about the program through seminars. A Bullying Prevention Coordinating Committee is organized and program implementation is planned. The coordinating committee includes all levels of school staff, as well as parents and students. An important aspect is strict supervision at the places and times in which bullying frequently occurs based on the student questionnaire. Not only are parents on the committee, but also all parents are asked to support the program through regular events and letters.[76]

DISCUSSION

As child and adolescent psychiatrists, we are in a unique position to propose and support effective prevention models that intervene in the developmental trajectory that results in youth violence. Involvement with the community as partners and strategy developers also has considerable value to ensure that the local needs assessment is authentic and that there is local/community support for the interventions.[80]

Programs such as those reviewed demonstrate that violence prevention is possible, but we need to muster the political and societal will to implement such programs for all children and youth everywhere. As health practitioners, child and adolescent psychiatrists are generally used for tertiary intervention and prevention. However, with strong roots in human development, we are in a unique position to advance primary and secondary prevention and influence elements that impact prevention at a primordial level. As our knowledge improves of the social determinants of health and factors that lead to a collective impact on well-being, we can better inform policy makers and community leaders on how to legislate laws with a strong public health approach to health promotion.[81] Physicians and health practitioners can play an important role in the primordial prevention arena by influencing policy on a broader level that reduces those factors that directly or indirectly work against well-being. The College of Physicians and Surgeons of Canada described the role of physicians as health advocates: "As Health Advocates, physicians responsibly use their expertise and influence to advance the health and well-being of individual patients, communities, and populations."[82] We can do so by becoming involved as the technical experts on boards of city council, state government, and national organizations.[83]

REFERENCES

1. Centers for Disease Control and Prevention, National Center for Injury Prevention and Control. 2010. Web based Injury Statistics Query and Reporting System

(WISQARS). Available at: http://www.cdc.gov/injury/wisqars/pdf/10LCID_Unintentional_Deaths_2010-a.pdf. Accessed August 12, 2015.

2. National Center for Injury Prevention and Control, Causes of injury death highlighting violence. Available at: cdc.gov/injury/wisqars/pdf/leading_causes_of_injury_death_highlighting_violence_2012-a.pdf. Accessed August 12, 2015.

3. Centers for Disease Control and Prevention. WISQARS, fatal injury reports, national and regional, 1999–2013. Available at: http://webappa.cdc.gov/sasweb/ncipc/mortrate10_us.html. Accessed August 12, 2015.

4. Eaton DK, Kann L, Kinchen S, et al, Centers for Disease Control and Prevention (CDC). Youth risk behavior surveillance—United States, 2011. MMWR Surveill Summ 2012;61(4):1–162. Available at: www.cdc.gov/mmwr/pdf/ss/ss6104.pdf. Accessed August 12, 2015.

5. Centers for Disease Control and Prevention. WISQARS, leading causes of nonfatal injury reports, 2001–2013. Available at: http://webappa.cdc.gov/sasweb/ncipc/nfilead2001.html. Accessed August 12, 2015.

6. Thornton TN, Craft CA, Dahlberg LL, et al. Best practices of youth violence prevention: a sourcebook for community action. Atlanta, GA: National Center for Injury Prevention, Centers of Disease Control and Prevention; 2002. Available at: www.cdc.gov/ncipc. Accessed November 24, 2015.

7. Kania J, Kramer M. Collective impact. Stanford Soc Innovat Rev 2011;9:36–41.

8. Dahlberg LL, Mercy JA. History of violence as a public health problem. Virtual Mentor 2009;11(2):167–72.

9. Krug EG, Dahlberg LL, Mercy JA, et al. World report on violence and health. Geneva (Switzerland): World Health Organization; 2002.

10. Maxfield MG, Widom CSP. The cycle of violence: revisited 6 years later. Arch Pediatr Adolesc Med 1996;150(4):390–5.

11. Widom CS, Maxfield MG. An update on the "cycle of violence". Washington, DC: U.S. Department of Justice, Office of Justice Programs; 2001.

12. Ford JD. Traumatic victimization in childhood and persistent problems with oppositional-defiance. In: Greenwald R, editor. Trauma and juvenile delinquency: theory, research, and interventions. Binghamton (NY): Haworth Maltreatment and Trauma Press/The Haworth Press, Inc; 2002. p. 25–58.

13. Margolin G, Gordis E. Children's exposure to violence in the family and community. Curr Dir Psychol Sci 2004;13(4):152–5.

14. Finkelhor D, Ormrod R, Turner H. Polyvictimization and trauma in a national longitudinal cohort. Dev Psychopathol 2007;19(1):149–66.

15. Finkelhor D, Ormrod R, Turner H. The developmental epidemiology of childhood victimization. J Interpers Violence 2009;24(5):711–31.

16. Al-Mateen CS, Webb SS, Sood AB. Predicting violence in public places. In: Sood AB, Cohen RO, editors. The Virginia Tech massacre: strategies and challenges for improving mental health policy on campus and beyond. New York: Oxford University Press; 2014. p. 127.

17. Garbarino J, Bradshaw CP, Vorrasi JA. Mitigating the effects of gun violence on children and youth. Future Child 2002;12(2):73–85.

18. Ratcliffe M, Ruddell M, Smith B. What is a "sense of foreshortened future?" A phenomenological study of trauma, trust, and time. Front Psychol 2014;5:1026.

19. Kelly DP, Erez E. Victim participation in the criminal justice system. In: Davis RC, Lurigio AJ, Skogan WG, editors. Victims of Crime. 2nd edition; 1997. p. 231–44.

20. Lansford JE, Miller-Johnson S, Berlin LJ, et al. Early physical abuse and later violent delinquency: a prospective longitudinal study. Child Maltreat 2007;12(3):233–45.

21. Teague R, Mazerolle P, Legosz M, et al. Linking childhood exposure to physical abuse and adult offending: examining mediating factors and gendered relationships. Justice Q 2008;25:313–48.
22. Felitti VJ, Anda RF, Nordenberg D, et al. Relationship of childhood abuse and household dysfunction to many of the leading causes of death in adults: the Adverse Childhood Experiences (ACE) study. Am J Prev Med 1998;14(4): 245–58.
23. Baglivio MT, Epps N, Swartz K, et al. The prevalence of adverse childhood experiences (ACE) in the lives of juvenile offenders. Journal of Juvenile Justice 2014; 3(2):1–23.
24. Fang X, Corso PS. Child maltreatment, youth violence, and intimate partner violence: developmental relationships. Am J Prev Med 2007;33(4):281–90.
25. Bell C, Fink P. Prevention of violence. In: Bell C, editor. Psychiatric aspects of violence: issues in prevention and treatment. San Francisco (CA): Jossey-Bass; 2000. p. 37–47.
26. Bell C, Flay B, Paikoff R. Strategies for health behavioral change. In: Chunn J, editor. The health behavioral change imperative: theory, education and practice in diverse populations. New York: Kluwer Academic/Plenum Publishers; 2002. p. 17–40.
27. Mihalic SW, Elliott DS. Short and long-term consequences of adolescent work. Youth Soc 1997;28(4):464–98.
28. Government Accountability Office (GAO). Residential programs: selected cases of death, abuse, and deceptive marketing. Washington, DC: US Government Accountability office; 2008.
29. Government Accountability Office (GAO). Residential facilities: state and federal oversight gaps may increase risk to youth well-being. Washington, DC: US Government Accountability office; 2008.
30. Chance S, Dickson D, Bennett PM, et al. Unlocking the doors: how fundamental changes in residential care can improve the ways we help children and families. Resid Treat Child Youth 2010;27(2):127–48.
31. Runyan CW. Using the Haddon matrix: introducing the third dimension. Inj Prev 1998;4(4):302–7.
32. Kitzman H, Olds DL, Henderson CR Jr, et al. Randomized trial of prenatal and infancy home visitation by nurses on the outcomes of pregnancy, dysfunctional caregiving, childhood injuries, and repeated childbearing among low-income women with no previous live births. JAMA 1997;278:644–52.
33. Eckenrode J, Campa M, Luckey DW, et al. Long-term effects of prenatal and infancy nurse home visitation on the life course of youths: 19-year follow-up of a randomized trial. Arch Pediatr Adolesc Med 2010;164:9–15.
34. Forgatch M, DeGarmo D. Parenting through change: an effective prevention program for single mothers. J Consult Clin Psychol 1999;67(5):711–24.
35. Forgatch MS, DeGarmo DS. Extending and testing the social interaction learning model with divorce samples. In: Reid JB, Patterson GR, Snyder J, editors. Antisocial behavior in children and adolescents: a developmental analysis and model for intervention. Washington, DC: American Psychological Association; 2002. p. 235–56.
36. Martinez C, Forgatch M. Preventing problems with boys' noncompliance: effects of a parent training intervention for divorcing mothers. J Consult Clin Psychol 2001;69(3):416–28.
37. Forgatch MS, Patterson GR, Degarmo DS, et al. Testing the Oregon delinquency model with 9-year follow-up of the Oregon Divorce Study. Dev Psychopathol 2009;21(02):637–60.

38. Tierney JP, Grossman JB, Resch NL. Making a difference: an impact study of big brothers/big sisters. Philadelphia: Public/Private Ventures; 1995.

39. Schwartz V. An overview of strategies to reduce school violence. ERIC/CUE Digest No. 115. New York: ERIC Clearinghouse on Urban Education; 1996. Available at: http://www.ericdigests.org/1998-1/overview.htm.

40. Karcher MJ. Connectedness and school violence: a framework for developmental interventions. In: Gerler E, editor. Handbook of school violence. Binghamton (NY): Haworth Press; 2004. p. 7–42.

41. Eby LT, Allen TD, Evans SC, et al. Does mentoring matter? A multidisciplinary meta-analysis comparing mentored and non-mentored individuals. J Vocat Behav 2008;72(2):254–67.

42. Herrera C. A first look into its potential. Philadelphia: Public/Private Ventures; 1999.

43. Henggeler SW, Rodick JD, Borduin CM, et al. Multisystemic treatment of juvenile offenders: effects on adolescent behavior and family interaction. Dev Psychol 1986;22:132–41.

44. Borduin CM, Henggeler SW, Blaske DM, et al. Multisystemic treatment of adolescent sexual offenders. Int J Offender Ther Comp Criminol 1990;35:105–14.

45. Borduin CM, Mann BJ, Cone LT, et al. Multisystemic treatment of serious juvenile offenders: long-term prevention of criminality and violence. J Consult Clin Psychol 1995;63:569–78.

46. Fain T, Greathouse SM, Turner SF, et al. Effectiveness of multisystemic therapy for minority youth: outcomes over 8 years in Los Angeles County. Journal of Juvenile Justice 2014;3(2):24–37.

47. Wagner DV, Borduin CM, Sawyer AM, et al. Long-term prevention of criminality in siblings of serious and violent juvenile offenders: a 25-year follow-up to a randomized clinical trial of multisystemic therapy. J Consult Clin Psychol 2014;82(3): 492–9.

48. Chamberlain P. Comparative evaluation of specialized foster care for seriously delinquent youths: a first step. Community Alternatives: International Journal for Family Care 1990;2:21–36.

49. Eddy J, Whaley R, Chamberlain P. The prevention of violent behavior by chronic and serious male juvenile offenders: a 2-year follow-up of a randomized clinical trial. J Emot Behav Disord 2004;12(1):2–8.

50. Chamberlain P, Leve LD, DeGarmo DS. Multidimensional treatment foster care for girls in the juvenile justice system: 2-year follow-up of a randomized clinical trial. J Consult Clin Psychol 2007;75(1):187–93.

51. Chamberlain P, Reid J. Comparison of two community alternatives to incarceration for chronic juvenile offenders. J Consult Clin Psychol 1998;5:857–63.

52. Gordon DA. Functional family therapy for delinquents. In: Ross RR, Antonowicz DH, Dhaliwal GK, editors. Going straight: effective delinquency prevention and offender rehabilitation. Ottawa (Canada): Air Training and Publications; 1995. p. 163–78.

53. Celinska K, Furrer S, Cheng C-C. An outcome-based evaluation of functional family therapy for youth with behavior problems. OJJDP Journal of Juvenile Justice 2013;2(2):23–36.

54. Aos S, Lee S, Drake E, et al. Return on investment: evidence-based options to improve statewide outcomes (Document No. 11-07-1201A). Olympia (Greece): Washington State Institute for Public Policy; 2011.

55. Hahn R, Fuqua-Whitley D, Wethington H, et al, Task Force on Community Preventive Services. Effectiveness of universal school-based programs to prevent

violence and aggressive behavior: a systematic review. Am J Prev Med 2007; 33(2 Suppl):S114–29.

56. Strawhacker MT. School violence: an overview. J Sch Nurs 2002;18(2):68–72.
57. Haynes NM, Emmons CL, Woodruff DW. School development program effects: linking implementation to outcomes [Special Issue: Changing Schools for Changing Times: The Comer School Development Program]. J Educ Stud Placed Risk 1998;3:71–85.
58. Mulvey EP, Cauffman E. The inherent limits of predicting school violence. Am Psychol 2001;56(10):797–802.
59. Newman KS, Fox C, Roth W, et al. Rampage: the social roots of school shootings. New York: Basic Books; 2004.
60. Langman P. Why kids kill–inside the minds of school shooters. New York: Palgrave Macmillan; 2009.
61. Levin J, Madfis E. Mass murder at school and cumulative strain: a sequential model. Am Behav Sci 2009;52(9):1227–45.
62. Nadel H, Spellmann M, Alvarez-Canino T, et al. The cycle of violence and victimization: a study of the school-based intervention of a multidisciplinary youth violence-prevention program. Am J Prev Med 1996;12(5 Suppl):109–19.
63. Bandura A. Social foundations of thought and action: a social cognitive theory. Englewood Cliffs (NJ): Prentice-Hall, Inc; 1986.
64. Dwyer K, Oher D, Warger C. Early warning, timely response: a guide to safe schools. Washington, DC: U.S. Department of Education; 1998.
65. Veltkamp LJ, Lawson A. Impact of trauma in school violence on the victim and perpetrator: a mental health perspective. In: Miller TW, editor. School violence and primary prevention. New York: Springer Science + Business Media; 2008. p. 185–200.
66. Callahan C. Threat assessment in school violence. In: Miller TW, editor. School violence and primary prevention. New York: Springer; 2008. p. 59–77.
67. Delizonna L, Alan I, Steiner HA. Case example of a school shooting: lessons learned in the wake of tragedy. In: Jimerson SR, Furlong MJ, editors. The handbook of school violence and school safety; from research to practice. Mahwah (NJ): Lawrence Erlbaum Associates; 2006. p. 617–29.
68. Greenberg MT, Kusche CA, Cook ET, et al. Promoting emotional competence in school-aged children: the effects of the PATHS curriculum. Dev Psychopathol 1995;7:117–36.
69. Kam C, Greenberg MT, Kusché CA. Sustained effects of the PATHS curriculum on the social and psychological adjustment of children in special education. J Emot Behav Disord 2004;12:66–78.
70. Curtis C, Norgate R. An evaluation of the promoting alternative thinking strategies curriculum at key stage 1. Educ Psychol Pract 2007;23:33–44.
71. Crean HF, Johnson DB. Promoting alternative thinking strategies (PATHS) and elementary school aged children's aggression: results from a cluster randomized trial. Am J Community Psychol 2013;52:56–72.
72. Botvin GJ, Epstein JA, Baker E, et al. School-based drug abuse prevention with inner-city youth. J Child Adolesc Subst Abuse 1997;6:5–19.
73. Botvin GJ, Baker E, Dusenbury L, et al. Preventing adolescent drug abuse through a multimodal cognitive-behavioral approach: results of a three-year study. J Consult Clin Psychol 1990;58:437–46.
74. Botvin GJ, Griffin KW, Diaz T, et al. Preventing illicit drug use in adolescents: long-term follow-up data from a randomized control trial of a school population. Addict Behav 2000;25:769–74.

75. Botvin GJ, Griffin KW, Nichols TR. Preventing youth violence and delinquency through a universal school-based prevention approach. Prev Sci 2006;7: 403–8.

76. Olweus D. Bullying among school children: intervention and prevention. In: Peters RD, McMahon RJ, Quinsey VL, editors. Aggression and violence throughout the life span. Newbury Park (CA): Sage Publications; 1992. p. 100–25.

77. Available at: http://www.blueprintsprograms.com/programResults.php. Accessed August 20, 2015.

78. Bauer NS, Lozano P, Rivara FP. The effectiveness of the Olweus bullying prevention program in public middle schools: a controlled trial. J Adolesc Health 2007; 40:266–74.

79. Schroeder BA, Messina A, Schroeder D, et al. The implementation of a statewide bullying prevention program preliminary findings from the field and the importance of coalitions. Health Promot Pract 2012;13(4):489–95.

80. Fleurence RL, Forsythe LP, Lauer M, et al. Engaging patients and stakeholders in research proposal review: the patient-centered outcomes research institute. Ann Intern Med 2014;161(2):122–30.

81. Secretary's advisory committee on health promotion and disease prevention objectives for 2010. Healthy People 2020: An Opportunity to Address the Societal Determinants of Health in the United States; 2010. Available at: http://www.healthypeople.gov/2010/hp2020/advisory/SocietalDeterminantsHealth.htm. Accessed July 26, 2010.

82. Public and Population Health. The Association of Faculties of Medicine of Canada Public Health Educators' Network. License: creative commons BY-NC-SA. p. 14. Available at: http://www.afmc-phprimer.ca. Accessed June 1, 2011.

83. Earnest MA, Wong SL, Federico SG. Perspective: physician advocacy: what is it and how do we do it? Acad Med 2010;85(1):63–7.

Empirically Based Strategies for Preventing Juvenile Delinquency

Dustin Pardini, PhD

KEYWORDS

- Juvenile delinquency • Prevention • Intervention • Crime

KEY POINTS

- Multiple causal factors have been implicated in the early emergence and persistence of serious conduct problems and delinquency in youth.
- In general, existing therapeutic interventions for youth showing antisocial behaviors tend to produce small to medium effects that are maintained over several years.
- Treatments that use cognitive-behavioral techniques (eg, parent management training, behavioral contracting, contingency management), and multimodal interventions seem to be most effective, particularly when administered to youth at highest risk for future delinquency.
- Peer group interventions are more effective with young children, and can produce iatrogenic effects when administered to adolescents who reinforce each other's antisocial behavior.
- Moving forward, there is a need to further develop comprehensive strategies to promote the widespread adoption of evidence-based practices designed to reduce juvenile delinquency within local communities and the juvenile justice system.

INTRODUCTION

Juvenile crime is a serious public health problem that exacts a significant financial and emotional toll on society.[1,2] Serious violence is particularly costly, with estimates suggesting that injuries and death caused by firearm violence costs the United States more than $70 billion annually.[2] Adolescents who engage in significant delinquent behavior are also at high risk for experiencing multiple deleterious outcomes in adulthood, including mental and physical health problems, unemployment, and relationship difficulties.[3] These factors have led policy makers and international health agencies to call for increased efforts to involve youth in interventions designed to prevent the

School of Criminology and Criminal Justice, Arizona State University, 411 North Central Avenue, Suite 600, Phoenix, AZ 85004, USA
E-mail address: dustin.pardini@asu.edu

Child Adolesc Psychiatric Clin N Am 25 (2016) 257–268
http://dx.doi.org/10.1016/j.chc.2015.11.009
1056-4993/16/$ – see front matter © 2016 Elsevier Inc. All rights reserved.

childpsych.theclinics.com

initiation and persistence of criminal behavior. This article discusses the existing research on the developmental course, cause, and prevention of delinquent behavior among children and adolescents.

DEVELOPMENTAL COURSE OF DELINQUENT BEHAVIOR

Population-based studies conducted across multiple countries and historical contexts have found that the prevalence and rate of criminal offending among youth tend to escalate during the teenage years then rapidly decrease across the 20s to early 30s.[4,5] However, there remains considerable heterogeneity in the developmental course of delinquent behavior within the population in terms of the onset, rate, and duration of offending. Over the past several decades, investigators have proposed various developmental models designed to delineate subgroups of youth who show distinct patterns of offending over time. One of the most enduring subtyping schemes is Moffitt's[6] developmental taxonomy model, which is founded on a large body of longitudinal research showing that there is a small portion of approximately 5% to 10% of youth who show severe conduct problems in childhood and who are at increased risk for showing criminal behavior into adulthood.[6] The criminal behavior of these childhood-onset cases (also referred to as life-course persistent offenders) is thought to be driven by a combination of early psychosocial adversity, a dysfunctional child-rearing environment, and subtle neurologic impairments. This pathway is in contrast with a larger group of youth who begin engaging in delinquent behaviors during adolescence. This group is thought to consist predominantly of oppositional adolescents who are poorly monitored and subsequently begin affiliating with deviant peers. Adolescent-onset offenders are posited to largely leave their antisocial ways behind during the transition into adulthood as they adopt prosocial roles (eg, stable job), spend less time with deviant peers, and engage in more mature decision making.

Over the past decade, a growing number of longitudinal studies have indicated that the developmental taxonomy model requires further revision.[7] For example, studies using latent trajectory group analysis have found that approximately 50% to 70% of youth who show severe conduct problems during childhood refrain from engaging in significant criminal offending during adolescence and young adulthood.[7,8] There is also substantial evidence that adolescent-onset offending is not as transient as was initially thought. Longitudinal studies have delineated a group of youth who show a rapid increase in offending during adolescence and continue engaging in criminal behavior well into adulthood.[7]

BEHAVIORAL PRECURSORS OF SEVERE DELINQUENT BEHAVIOR

Longitudinal studies have consistently found that early forms of problem behavior in childhood often precede the development of severe delinquent behavior during adolescence. Loeber[9] proposed a heuristic model based on longitudinal research describing a developmental progression of 3 overlapping, but distinct, subtypes of antisocial behavior (authority defiance, covert conduct problems, overt conduct problems). According to this model, intense, affectively laden conflicts with authority figures (eg, arguing, defiance, oppositional conflict) before school entry often proceed or co-occur with the development of more severe overt and covert conduct problems. Behaviors in the overt pathway tend to progress from minor acts of verbal and physical aggression (eg, threatening, bullying, hitting, teasing others) in childhood to acts of serious violence during adolescence (eg, murder, robbery, attacking with a weapon), whereas behaviors in the covert pathway progress from lying and minor theft (eg, shoplifting) beginning in childhood to more serious acts of theft (eg, burglary, auto theft) during adolescence. As outlined in detail later, developmentally appropriate and empirically validated intervention programs have been designed to target youth showing the range of problem behaviors that make up these pathways.

CAUSES OF JUVENILE DELINQUENCY

Contemporary developmental models of youth delinquency founded on longitudinal research have served as the foundation for the development targeted by intervention programs, such as the Biopsychosocial Model,[10] Developmental Taxonomy Model,[6] the Contextual Social-Cognitive Model,[11] and the Seattle Social Development Model.[12] Each of these models posits that early childhood dispositional characteristics coupled with an accumulating array of adverse sociocontextual risk factors serve to perpetuate early emerging and persistent delinquency. However, there are a myriad of different factors that have been linked to the development in delinquent behavior in longitudinal and cross-sectional studies.[6,13–15] **Box 1** provides some examples of these factors, which span multiple life domains.

What remains unclear is the extent to which various risk factors represent key causal mechanisms in the development of delinquent behavior, as opposed to spurious correlates. In addition, it has become increasingly evident that there are multiple causal pathways underlying the behavioral manifestations of antisocial behavior in youth, and these pathways involve complex mediating and moderating mechanisms. On a rudimentary level, longitudinal evidence suggests that, as youth begin accumulating a diverse array of risk factors across development, they become increasingly likely to engage in persistent antisocial behavior.[16–18] For example, children born with significant emotional and behavioral regulation problems who are exposed to disadvantaged and maladaptive sociocontextual environments (eg, poor neighborhoods, harsh parenting) are at particularly high risk for developing severe conduct problems in early childhood.[19] These children tend to enter school with poor social and academic skills, leading to aggressive conflicts with both peers and teachers.[20] Over time, they may increasingly experience academic failure and become rejected by mainstream peers, which can result in an increased affiliation with deviant youth who reinforce antisocial behaviors and beliefs.[10] As adolescents, these youth may then become further attached to a life of crime by developing substance use problems and coming into contact with the juvenile justice system.

MULTITIERED APPROACHES TO DELINQUENCY PREVENTION

Using etiologic models as a guide, several delinquency prevention programs have been developed to target a diverse array of risk factors thought to perpetuate antisocial behavior at different stages of development. These programs can be classified into 4 tiers based on the characteristics of the targeted youth and overarching goal of the intervention.

- Primary prevention: Programs designed to reduce the overall prevalence of risk factors for delinquency within the general population.
- Selective prevention: Interventions that target children exposed to early sociocontextual risk factors associated with delinquency (eg, poverty, teenage pregnancy).
- Indicated prevention: Programs that target youth showing predelinquent conduct problems to prevent them from engaging in serious crime.
- Therapeutic interventions: Treatments that target youth showing delinquent behavior to promote desistance from criminal offending.

Box 1
Examples of risk factors commonly implicated in the development of severe and persistent delinquent behavior

Sociodemographic factors
Family poverty
Teenage mother
Single parent
Dispositional factors
Dysregulated anger
Fearlessness/sensation seeking
Lack of empathy/guilt
Hyperactive/impulsive
Peer factors
Affiliation with antisocial peers
Peer rejection/victimization
School factors
Low school motivation/bonding
Academic failure
Parenting factors
Low positive reinforcement
Low supervision/monitoring
High parent-child conflict
Abuse and neglect
Lack of clearly defined rules
Inconsistent discipline
Low parental warmth/involvement

Family factors
Family history of crime
High family conflict
Parental mental health problems
Intimate partner violence
Neighborhood factors
Neighborhood poverty/crime
Social-cognitive factors
Poor social problem-solving skills
Positive expectations for aggression
Values favoring delinquency
Hostile attributional bias
Psychophysiologic factors
Low resting heart rate
Poor aversive conditioning
Neurocognitive factors
Low intelligence
Poor executive control
Poor response reversal learning
Affective processing deficits
Neurobiological factors
Low limbic reactivity to distress cues

Because of space considerations, the remainder of this article reviews research on effective indicated prevention programs and therapeutic interventions targeting youth at highest risk for engaging in severe and persistent criminal behavior.

GENERAL CHARACTERISTICS OF EFFECTIVE PROGRAMS

On average, existing indicated prevention and therapeutic intervention programs have been found to produce small to medium effects on conduct problems and delinquent behavior.[21–23] The effectiveness of these programs does not seem to systematically vary as a function of the participants' age, gender, and race/ethnicity.[21–23] However, there is tremendous heterogeneity in the effectiveness of various programs. Recent meta-analytical studies have provided some insights into the characteristics of the most effective interventions.[21–23]

- Interventions that have well-defined protocols and include regular fidelity checks to ensure services are being delivered in an appropriate manner tend to be more effective.
- Interventions focused on therapeutic approaches (eg, mentoring programs, parent management training, contingency management) are more effective than those that use external control techniques (eg, boot camps, intensive supervision).
- Treatments that use cognitive-behavioral strategies (eg, parent management training, behavioral contracting, contingency management) and multimodal interventions seem to produce larger behavioral improvements.
- Therapeutic interventions implemented with highly delinquent youth tend to produce larger effects than indicated prevention programs with youth showing less severe behavior problems.

- Peer group interventions tend to be more effective in younger children, and can produce iatrogenic effects in older youth if they are allowed to reinforce each other's antisocial behavior.

COMMON COMPONENTS OF EVIDENCE-BASED PROGRAMS

The most widely adopted and rigorously evaluated programs designed to prevent or reduce delinquent behavior have been developed and evaluated within academic settings. **Table 1** presents some name-brand manualized programs that regularly appear on vetted lists of empirically supported interventions for antisocial and delinquent youth.[24,25] Some core elements found in 1 or more of these programs are reviewed later.

Parent Management Training

Parenting management training uses cognitive-behavioral treatment strategies to disrupt preexisting coercive cycles of parent-child conflict that reinforce noncompliance and equip parents with effective behavioral management techniques based on principles of operant conditioning. These programs typically focus on increasing parents' use of positive reinforcement, warmth/involvement, effective discipline, and proactive monitoring, while reducing their use of harsh and abusive discipline. A combination of didactic instruction, modeling, and in-session role plays are typically used to teach specific techniques. Parents are then given weekly practice assignments to facilitate the application of newly learned skills to real-life situations. Some programs provide in-vivo coaching during parent-child interactions to ensure that caretakers are appropriately implementing specific skills.

Behavioral Contracting

This is a positive-reinforcement intervention that is widely used to modify maladaptive behavior. Parents (and sometimes teachers) are trained to develop a clearly outlined plan for systematically tracking youth behavior (eg, home-school behavior report cards). Privileges and other rewards are then earned by youth as they complete scheduled activities and fulfill behavioral goals. Caretakers and youth often work together to formulate the specific contingencies outlined in the behavioral contract. Token economies and level systems are commonly used to index behavioral progress.

Socioemotional and Problem-Solving Skills Training

These cognitive-behavioral interventions are typically implemented with preschool and elementary school children in small group settings. Sessions are used to teach skills involving objectively evaluating peaceful conflict resolution, anger management, impulse control, goal-setting, social problem solving, friendship building, coping with teasing and peer pressure, and emotional perspective taking. These skills are practiced, refined, and reinforced in sessions using a diverse array of strategies, including hypothetical vignettes, role plays, and skits. Children are often assigned tasks to be completed between sessions in which they apply newly learned skills to real-life interpersonal situations of increasing complexity. In addition, youth are often asked to identify weekly behavioral goals that are monitored by parents and teachers. These goals are reviewed at each session, and rewards are often given for accomplishing set goals.

Table 1
Examples of empirically supported programs designed to prevent the development of severe and persistent delinquent behavior

Program	Target Population	Intervention Strategy
Parent-child interaction therapy[26]	Children aged 2–6 y showing severe oppositional/defiant behaviors	Parent-Child Interaction Therapy is a parent-focused intervention that is implemented in the context of naturalistic play settings between the parent and child in which a therapist provides guidance behind a one-way mirror through the use of a hidden ear device worn by the parent. This technique provides the parent with the unique opportunity to practice and master skills in vivo rather than passively learning through didactic interactions with the therapist. Sessions focus on strengthening the parent-child relationship through child-directed play, reinforcing positive behaviors, and decreasing maladaptive behaviors through the use of consistently implemented behavioral management techniques
The Incredible Years Program[27]	Children aged 4–7 y diagnosed with ODD or CD	The core intervention includes both a parent and child component. The child component consists of groups of 6 or 7 children who attend weekly 2-h sessions for approximately 17 wk. Videotaped vignettes and life-sized puppets are used to promote emotional empathy, perspective-taking skills, conflict resolution skills, anger regulation, and friendship building. The parent training intervention consists of approximately 22 sessions that use videotapes to model appropriate ways to deal with problematic parent-child interactions. Sessions address topics such as promoting effective play techniques, limit setting, handling misbehavior, and the communication of emotions
Problem-solving skills training with parent management training[28]	Children aged 10–13 y diagnosed with ODD or CD	This program mainly comprises 12 weekly sessions (30–50 min each) designed to teach and reinforce strategies for effectively dealing with interpersonal conflicts. As part of these sessions, children are taught to objectively evaluate problem situations, develop prosocial goals, and generate alternative solutions to meet their goals. Children initially practice these skills using hypothetical conflict situations that may arise in the settings in which they are having the most problems. Children are then assigned supersolver tasks in which they apply these strategies to real-life situations. The parent management training portion of the intervention involves a core set of 12 weekly sessions (45–60 min each) designed to teach parents to use behavioral principles to modify problematic child behavior. Topics covered in sessions include the appropriate use of parenting techniques such as positive reinforcement, time out, verbal reprimands, negotiation, and behavioral contracting. Therapists also help parents identify explicit school goals, which are monitored using a home-school behavioral report card system, and children are rewarded for achieving specific behavioral milestones

MST (Multisystemic Therapy)[29]	Delinquent adolescents aged 11–17 y	MST emphasizes the interaction between adolescents and the multiple environmental systems that influence their behavior (eg, peers, family, school, community). MST is delivered in the family's natural environment and can include a combination of different treatment approaches (eg, parent management training, family therapy, school consultation) tailored to the needs of the family. Treatment strategies are developed in collaboration with family members after identifying factors that help maintain the adolescents' deviant behavior. Methods for overcoming barriers to positive behavior change are also discussed in session. Clinicians are guided by a set of 9 MST principles, which include concepts like focusing on strengths and encouraging responsible behavior
Multidimensional treatment foster care[30]	Delinquent adolescents aged 12–17 y	Multidimensional treatment foster care was designed as an alternative to traditional group care for delinquent adolescents (aged 12–17 y) removed from their homes. This multicomponent intervention places youth with a community-based foster family, where contingencies governing the youth's behavior are modified through consultation with a comprehensive treatment team. Each foster family is assigned a program supervisor, foster parent consultant, behavior support specialist, family therapist, parent daily report caller, and consulting psychiatrist to assist with program implementation. Adolescents earn privileges through a level system by following a daily program of scheduled activities and fulfilling behavioral expectations. Program staff provide around-the-clock support for crisis management, assist in creating a school-based support plan, and provide individualized skills coaching as necessary. The adolescents' future guardians assist in treatment planning, engage in family therapy, and begin applying newly learned parenting skills during home visits
FFT (Functional Family Therapy)[31]	Delinquent adolescents aged 11–17 y	FFT is an intervention for delinquent adolescents (aged 11–17 y) and their families that combines principles of family systems theory with cognitive-behavioral approaches. FFT consists of 3 intervention phases: (1) engagement/motivation, (2) behavior change, and (3) generalization. During the engagement/motivation phase, the therapist begins establishing a strong therapeutic alliance with the family, addresses maladaptive family beliefs to increase expectations for change, and reduces negativity and blaming within the family system. The behavior change phase involves implementing an individualized treatment plan to improve family functioning, which may include building relational skills, enhancing positive parenting, and reducing maladaptive familial interactions. In addition, the generalization phase is designed to improve the family's ability to competently influence the systems in which it is embedded (eg, school, community, justice system) in order to maintain positive behavioral change. Families in FFT typically attend 12 treatment sessions over the course of 3–4 mo

Abbreviations: CD, conduct disorder; ODD, oppositional defiant disorder.
Data from Refs.[26–31]

Family Therapy

Interventions involving family therapy are most often used with adolescents showing serious delinquent behavior. These programs typically bring together family members to identify maladaptive behaviors, beliefs, and interaction styles that serve to perpetuate youth antisocial behavior. Individualized treatment plans are developed to improve family functioning, which may include building relational skills, enhancing positive parenting, and reducing maladaptive familial interactions. These programs often help families learn how to effectively leverage systems and resources in the community in order to promote and maintain reductions in youth antisocial behavior.

Case Management Services

Some intensive programs provide case management services designed to help families obtain an array of services based on an individualized treatment plan. This assistance can involve coordinating the activities of members of a larger treatment team (eg, consulting psychiatrist, behavioral specialist), providing crisis intervention services, advocating on behalf of families as they navigate various systems of care, and working with families to develop an aftercare plan.

PHARMACOTHERAPY

The extent to which psychotropic medications may help to reduce serious conduct problems and delinquent behavior remains unclear. Randomized placebo studies investigating the effectiveness of specific medications tend to be small and none have extended follow-ups. However, some accumulating evidence suggests that methylphenidate may help reduce aggression in youth with comorbid attention-deficit/hyperactivity disorder (ADHD) and severe conduct problems,[32] with decreased appetite and insomnia being the most commonly reported side effects. Similar effects have been reported in randomized trials involving the antipsychotic risperidone, although side effects such as lethargy, headaches, and weight gain are a concern.[33] A more recent randomized controlled trial found that risperidone may be an effective adjunctive therapy for aggressive youth with ADHD and oppositional defiant disorder/conduct disorder who continue to show behavioral impairments after receiving parent management training and stimulant treatment.[34] Based on this research, it is recommended that psychosocial interventions be considered the first line of treatment of youth who show severe conduct problems, with stimulant medications being used when comorbid ADHD is present, and risperidone being considered as a potential adjunct for youth showing treatment-resistant aggression and conduct problems.

PROMOTING THE WIDESPREAD ADOPTION OF EVIDENCE-BASED PRACTICES

Over the past decade, there have been considerable efforts to disseminate several name-brand delinquency prevention programs across the country. Companies have been formed to provide certification training and supporting program materials. This effort has resulted in several independent studies examining the effectiveness of various programs in real-world settings. Many of these investigations have found small or nonsignificant treatment effects on conduct problems when comparing name-brand programs with usual care, which seems to be in part caused by reduced adherence to treatment protocols.[35] Moreover, it is increasingly recognized that the adoption and maintenance of evidence-based programs requires active support and engagement by policy makers and shareholders in the community and juvenile justice system. Taken together, this emphasizes the importance of building the support and infrastructure needed to incorporate evidence-based practices designed to reduce juvenile delinquency in real-world settings. Two recently developed initiatives designed to accomplish this task are outlined later.

Communities That Care

The overarching goal of the Communities that Care (CTC) initiative is to (1) improve collaborative action across community stakeholders; (2) promote community-wide values and beliefs that are intolerant of youth delinquency; and (3) increase the adoption of sustainable evidence-based programs that reduce known risk factors associated with delinquency and related problem behavior.[36] As part of the program, school-wide surveys are administered to assess the overall level of specific risk factors associated with delinquent behavior present among youth living in the community. Community stakeholders are then trained to select and implement specific programs that have been shown to reduce the predominant risk factors among youth living in the community. Evidence from a large randomized controlled trial suggests that the CTC program is a cost-effective strategy for preventing the onset of delinquency and substance use among adolescents.[37] However, this initial trial focused primarily on the adoption of universal prevention programs, and it may prove difficult for community stakeholders to implement a greater array of interventions that are specifically designed for youth showing serious conduct problems and delinquent behavior.

Standardized Program Evaluation Protocol

Over the past several years, juvenile justice agencies have increasingly attempted to increase the adoption of evidence-based practices using the Standardized Program Evaluation Protocol (SPEP) rating scale.[38] This instrument assesses the extent to which existing programs are using practices that have been associated with reduced recidivism in meta-analytical research. The benefit of this approach is that it places name-brand and generic local programs on a common metric for comparison, and provides agencies with clear information about how existing programs can be improved to increase their adherence to evidence-based practices. A recent evaluation of the SPEP system conducted in 5 Arizona counties found preliminary evidence supporting the utility of the measure for indexing program effectiveness.[39] More rigorous examinations of the SPEP system over the coming years will be critical in determining its ultimate value in helping to enhance the adoption of evidence-based practices and reduce juvenile delinquency.

SUMMARY

There are now several well-defined and empirically supported interventions that are effective at reducing severe conduct problems and delinquent behavior in youth. However, these programs tend to produce modest behavioral gains, and many youth continue to show significant antisocial behavior at the end of treatment. If interventions can be better tailored to the unique characteristics of children based on the developmental mechanisms underlying their conduct problems, more pronounced and sustained treatment effects are likely to be achieved. Efforts are currently underway to modify existing treatments to target the unique causal factors underlying the behavior problems of subgroups of antisocial youth.[40] These ongoing innovations coupled with recent efforts to integrate multitiered evidence-based practices into real-world settings hold great promise for reducing the prevalence of severe and persistent delinquent behavior among youth.

REFERENCES

1. Welsh BC, Loeber R, Stevens BR, et al. Costs of juvenile crime in urban areas: a longitudinal perspective. Youth Violence Juv Justice 2008;6(1):3–27.
2. Corso PS, Mercy JA, Simon TR, et al. Medical costs and productivity losses due to interpersonal and self-directed violence in the United States. Am J Prev Med 2007;32(6):474–82.
3. Costello EJ, Maughan B. Annual research review: optimal outcomes of child and adolescent mental illness. J Child Psychol Psychiatry 2015;56(3):324–41.
4. Loeber R, Farrington DP, Stouthamer-Loeber M, et al. Violence and serious theft: development and prediction from childhood to adulthood. New York: Routledge; 2008.
5. Farrington DP. Age and crime. In: Tonry M, Morris N, editors. Crime and justice: an annual review of research, vol. 7. Chicago: University of Chicago Press; 1986. p. 189–250.
6. Moffitt TE. Life-course persistent versus adolescence-limited antisocial behavior. In: Cicchetti D, Cohen DJ, editors. Developmental psychopathology. 2nd edition. New York: Wiley; 2006. p. 570–98.
7. Fairchild G, van Goozen SH, Calder AJ, et al. Research review: evaluating and reformulating the developmental taxonomic theory of antisocial behaviour. J Child Psychol Psychiatry 2013;54(9):924–40.
8. Odgers CL, Moffitt TE, Broadbent JM, et al. Female and male antisocial trajectories: from childhood origins to adult outcomes. Dev Psychopathol 2008;20(2): 673–716.
9. Loeber R. Natural histories of conduct problems, delinquency, and associated substance use: evidence for developmental progressions. Adv Clin Child Psychol 1988;11:73–124.
10. Dodge KA, Pettit GS. A biopsychosocial model of the development of chronic conduct problems in adolescence. Dev Psychol 2003;39(2):349–71.
11. Lochman JE, Wells KC. Contextual social-cognitive mediators and child outcome: a test of the theoretical model in the coping power program. Dev Psychopathol 2002;14(4):945–67.
12. Catalano RF, Hawkins JD. The social development model: a theory of antisocial behavior. In: Hawkins JD, editor. Delinquency and crime: current theories. New York: Cambridge University Press; 1996. p. 149–97.
13. Loeber R, Pardini D. Neurobiology and the development of violence: common assumptions and controversies. In: Hodgins S, Viding E, Plodowski A, editors. The neurobiological basis of violence: science and rehabilitation. Oxford (United Kingdom): Oxford University Press; 2009. p. 1–22.
14. Assink M, van der Put CE, Hoeve M, et al. Risk factors for persistent delinquent behavior among juveniles: a meta-analytic review. Clin Psychol Rev 2015;42:47–61.
15. Farrington DP. Prospective longitudinal research on the development of offending. Aust New Zeal J Criminol 2015;48(3):314–35.
16. Atzaba-Poria N, Pike A, Deater-Deckard K. Do risk factors for problem behaviour act in a cumulative manner? An examination of ethnic minority and majority children through an ecological perspective. J Child Psychol Psychiatry 2004;45(4):707–18.
17. Loeber R, Pardini D, Homish DL, et al. The prediction of violence and homicide in young men. J Consult Clin Psychol 2005;73(6):1074–88.
18. Stouthamer-Loeber M, Loeber R, Wei E, et al. Risk and promotive effects in the explanation of persistent serious delinquency in boys. J Consult Clin Psychol 2002;70(1):111–23.

19. Moffitt TE, Caspi A. Childhood predictors differentiate life-course persistent and adolescence-limited antisocial pathways among males and females. Dev Psychopathol 2001;13(2):355–75.

20. Dodge KA, Greenberg MT, Malone PS. Testing an idealized dynamic cascade model of the development of serious violence in adolescence. Child Dev 2008; 79(6):1907–27.

21. Sawyer AM, Borduin CM, Dopp AR. Long-term effects of prevention and treatment on youth antisocial behavior: a meta-analysis. Clin Psychol Rev 2015;42: 130–44.

22. Lipsey MW. The primary factors that characterize effective interventions with juvenile offenders: a meta-analytic overview. Vict Offender 2009;4(2):124–47.

23. Vries SL, Hoeve M, Assink M, et al. Practitioner review: effective ingredients of prevention programs for youth at risk of persistent juvenile delinquency–recommendations for clinical practice. J Child Psychol Psychiatry 2015;56(2):108–21.

24. Eyberg SM, Nelson MM, Boggs SR. Evidence-based psychosocial treatments for children and adolescents with disruptive behavior. J Clin Child Adolesc Psychol 2008;37(1):215–37.

25. Office of the Surgeon General. Youth violence: a report of the surgeon general. Rockville (MD): Office of the Surgeon General; 2001. Available at: http://www. ncbi.nlm.nih.gov/books/NBK44294/. Accessed December 30, 2015.

26. Eyberg SM, Boggs SR, Algina J. Parent-child interaction therapy: a psychosocial model for the treatment of young children with conduct problem behavior and their families. Psychopharmacol Bull 1995;31(1):83–91.

27. Webster-Stratton C, Reid MJ, Hammond M. Treating children with early-onset conduct problems: intervention outcomes for parent, child, and teacher training. J Clin Child Adolesc Psychol 2004;33(1):105–24.

28. Kazdin AE. Problem-solving skills training and parent management training for oppositional defiant disorder and conduct disorder. Evidence-based psychotherapies for children and adolescents. 2nd edition. New York: Guilford Press; 2010. p. 211–26.

29. Henggeler SW. Efficacy studies to large-scale transport: the development and validation of multisystemic therapy programs. Annu Rev Clin Psychol 2011;7: 351–81.

30. Chamberlain P. The Oregon Multidimensional Treatment Foster Care Model: features, outcomes, and progress in dissemination. Cogn Behav Pract 2003;10: 303–12.

31. Sexton TL. Functional family therapy in clinical practice: an evidence-based treatment model for working with troubled adolescents. New York: Routledge; 2010.

32. Pappadopulos E, Woolston S, Chait A, et al. Pharmacotherapy of aggression in children and adolescents: efficacy and effect size. J Can Acad Child Adolesc Psychiatry 2006;15:27–39.

33. Loy JH, Merry SN, Hetrick SE, et al. Atypical antipsychotics for disruptive behaviour disorders in children and youths. Cochrane Database Syst Rev 2012;(9):CD008559.

34. Aman MG, Bukstein OG, Gadow KD, et al. What does risperidone add to parent training and stimulant for severe aggression in child attention-deficit/hyperactivity disorder? J Am Acad Child Adolesc Psychiatry 2014;53(1):47–60.e41.

35. Pardini DA, Pasalich DS, Kimonis ER, et al. Conduct disorder. Gabbard's treatments of psychiatric disorders. 5th edition. Arlington (VA): American Psychiatric Publishing; 2014. p. 739–46.

36. Hawkins JD, Catalano RF, Arthur MW. Promoting science-based prevention in communities. Addict Behav 2002;27(6):951–76.

37. Kuklinski MR, Fagan AA, Hawkins JD, et al. Benefit-cost analysis of a randomized evaluation of Communities that Care: monetizing intervention effects on the initiation of delinquency and substance use through grade 12. J Exp Criminol 2015; 11:1–28.
38. Lipsey MW, Howell JC. A broader view of evidence-based programs reveals more options for state juvenile justice systems. Criminol Publ Pol 2012;11(3): 515–23.
39. Lipsey MW. The Arizona Standardized Program Evaluation Protocol (SPEP) for assessing the effectiveness of programs for juvenile probationers. Nashville (TN): Vanderbilt University Center for Evaluation Research and Methodology; 2008.
40. Hawes DJ, Price MJ, Dadds MR. Callous-unemotional traits and the treatment of conduct problems in childhood and adolescence: a comprehensive review. Clin Child Fam Psychol Rev 2014;17:248–67.

Child Obesity and Mental Health: A Complex Interaction

Leigh Small, PhD, RN, CPNP-PC[a],*, Alexis Aplasca, MD[b]

KEYWORDS

- Childhood obesity • Internalizing • Externalizing • Depression • Anxiety
- Body image • Self-esteem • Weight bias

KEY POINTS

- Both mental health and weight-based challenges are pervasive in America's youth.
- Child obesity and mental health treatment strategies share many common elements.
- A wide variety of intervention strategies is needed to make an impact on the comorbid problems of child obesity and psychosocial disturbances.
- Addressing both mental wellness and obesity from a healthy-lifestyle approach appears to be both feasible and effective and requires interprofessional collaboration.
- Broad-based conceptualization of these issues is necessary for strategically aligned intervention that should occur at the individual, family, organizational, community, and policy levels.

The upsurge in the US national prevalence and incidence rates of childhood obesity ($\geq$95th age- and gender-specific body mass index [BMI] percentile) over the last 3 decades has led to childhood obesity being considered a health epidemic.[1,2] The increased prevalence of child and adolescent obesity is unfortunately not a uniquely American phenomenon because its effects have been noted in many countries.[3–5] As a result of the increased frequency with which child obesity presents clinically and the focused worldwide attention, associated health conditions have become more evident, one of which is the coexistence of obesity and mental health problems. A survey of the literature dating back to 1995 reveals an increasing number of research publications related to comorbid psychiatric and psychological conditions and

Commercial or Financial Disclosure and Funding Statements: Neither Drs L. Small or A. Aplasca have any commercial or financial conflicts of interest to disclose that may affect the content of this publication. There were no funding sources used to support the development of this article.
[a] Family and Community Health Nursing Department, Virginia Commonwealth University School of Nursing, 1100 East Leigh Street, PO Box 980567, Richmond, VA 23298, USA;
[b] Pediatrics and Psychiatry, Children's Hospital of Richmond/Virginia Treatment Center for Children, Virginia Commonwealth University School of Medicine, 515 North 10th Street, Richmond, VA 23298, USA
* Corresponding author.
E-mail address: LSmall2@VCU.edu

childhood obesity. Much of the research has focused on the temporal connection of obesity and mental health problems in children as well as developing and rigorously testing interventions that are both developmentally informed and condition-specific.

The mental health aspects of obesity are broad with respect to specific psychiatric diagnoses and the psychological and psychosocial effects and include body image disturbances, low self-esteem, social stigma/impaired social relationships, weight-based victimization, low health-related quality of life, depressive symptoms, risk for disordered eating (binge eating, loss of control eating, eating in the absence of hunger), high levels of anxiety and internalizing (depression and anxiety), and externalizing behavioral problems (hyperactivity and aggressiveness).[6–10]

PREDICTORS OF LATER LIFE OBESITY

The predictive relationship of obesity and psychosocial disturbances and vice versa has been widely disputed in the research literature, although several psychological variables have been found to significantly predict later obesity or a worsening of obesity in children. For example, studies have independently identified internalizing (ie, depression) and externalizing (ie, hyperactivity, aggression) behaviors at ages 5 and 8 years, respectively, as predictors of obesity in older teens and young adults (18–23 years)[11,12] and later adulthood (30 and 34 years).[13] A secondary data analysis of the large British Cohort Study dataset replicated these findings.[14] In this study, teacher- and parent-reported child psychological functioning at 5 and 10 years of age was tested as predictors of obesity at 30 and 34 years of age. The findings suggest childhood hyperactivity and inattention place a person at increased risk for obesity later in life.[14]

Several researchers have investigated the predictive association of depression to later obesity.[13] Many study findings support the hypothesis that depression is an independent predictor of obesity[15,16]; however, this finding has been disputed by other researchers recently.[17,18] Thus, it appears that the predictive contribution of depression (an internalizing behavior) in early childhood to later life obesity is yet unclear; however, young child externalizing behaviors (eg, hyperactivity, aggressiveness, and inattentiveness) seem to have predictive relevance.

CHILDHOOD OBESITY AS A PREDICTOR OF IMPAIRED PSYCHOSOCIAL HEALTH

Impairment in psychosocial functioning is much broader in scope than psychiatric impairment. Despite not meeting the threshold for specific psychiatric diagnoses, psychological consequences of child obesity are significant. Negative self-body image, bullying and weight-biased peer interactions, negative school experiences, medical comorbidities, aberrant or promiscuous sexual behavior, substance abuse, and other negative health-related behaviors disrupt the psychosocial development of a child.

Childhood obesity is associated with behavior problems when girls start school. At this early age, there already appears to be gender differences because obese boys are not similarly affected.[6] In contrast to some commonly held beliefs, excess body weight status in early childhood does not predict the onset of new internalizing or externalizing behavior problems during the first 2 years of school.[19] However, as children mature and experience increased peer and adult interactions, perception of their personal weight status and the reaction to their weight status influence their self-perceptions. Wang and colleagues[20] conducted a cross-sectional secondary data analysis, which found that obesity in 10- and 11-year-old children independently predicted self-esteem 2 and 4 years later with obese children significantly more likely than normal-weight children to report low self-esteem 4 years later (odds ratio = 1.82; 95% confidence interval: 1.01–3.78).

A child's development of self-image and self-perception is difficult to study. Collectively, the studies of young obese children aged 5 to 13 years raise the following questions:

a. Do very young children have a limited perception of their own weight status in relation to the weight of other similarly aged children?
b. Do young children have limited insight regarding how one's weight status may influence the attitudes and behaviors of others (peers and adults)?
c. Do young children have the ability for abstract thinking to self-reflect or have a self-perception related to their weight and articulate this to others?; or
d. Do researchers have the capability to measure these complex variables across children in this age range?

Whether the collective research findings appropriately represent the development of psychosocial sequelae obese children experience over time or if there is inherent measurement error related to young children's limited abilities to express complex thoughts (ie, self-esteem, body image), it should be noted that many of these studies are cross-sectional in design or are secondary analyses of existing datasets. Overall, there is a low level of evidence on the subject.

Children who are larger than average have been found to be at elevated risk for interpersonal and intrapersonal problems.[16,21] The research team of Cui et al[22] reported that BMI significantly predicted lower health-related quality of life, a finding confirmed by other researchers,[23–26] particularly in the case of prepubertal children and those in early adolescence. Obesity in preadolescent youth has been found to be predictive of bullying or weight-based victimization.[27,28] Although victimization is not a psychological sequelae of obesity per se, it is associated with many psychological consequences.

The developmental stage of adolescence is associated with increased risk-taking behavior, impulsivity, and other environmental factors, coinciding with the top 3 causes of teen death in the United States, which are consistently reported to be accidents, homicide, and suicide. The Youth Risk Behavior Survey conducted by the US Centers of Disease Control and Prevention provides epidemiologic data regarding high school–aged children throughout the country, reporting on several known high-risk behaviors, such as substance use, sexual activity, and suicidality.[29] These high-risk behaviors have also been extrapolated to predict maladaptive health behaviors, such as those linked with obesity and other medical and psychiatric conditions in adulthood.

Studies looking at the developmental trajectory of obese adolescents have suggested an increased likelihood of repeating a grade and less expectation of going to college. Loneliness, increased peer pressure to use substances, engagement in delinquent activities, low quality of life, and higher age at dating initiation have also been reported.[30] Increased rates of completed suicide in obese adolescents appear to occur at similar rates to their age-matched normal-weight peers,[31] although being obese or extremely obese has been associated with engagement in suicidal ideation and behavior.[32] Chronic suicidal thoughts and behaviors are risk factors for future completed suicide, but studies drawing this conclusion in obese children are not yet available.

Childhood obesity is linked with several chronic physical health conditions, such as metabolic syndrome, type 2 diabetes, hypertension, dyslipidemia, disordered sleep, and orthopedic problems.[2,5,6,33] Although studies have shown a relationship between psychosocial distress in young people with obesity, those who experience obesity-related physical health conditions have additional risk factors for the development of psychopathology due in part to disease chronicity. Understanding these associations is an important public health issue, as higher rates of psychiatric diagnoses are associated with poorer adherence to medical treatment of both psychiatric and physical health problems.[34]

The interrelationships that exist between child obesity and psychosocial disturbances are complex and appear to differ by child age; however, the importance of recognizing the psychosocial risks that obese children of all ages face has important implications. In a retrospective study by Janicke and colleagues,[35] one-third of children and adolescents with an obesity-related health condition had a comorbid internalizing or externalizing disorder, compared with the 1 in 5 children in the general population. These and similar findings underscore the need to treat a child's obesity to reduce risk for other physical health sequelae, to regularly conduct screenings for psychosocial and mental health difficulties, and initiate interventions that address all aspects early on as a comprehensive approach to treatment.

PSYCHIATRIC COMORBIDITIES OF OBESITY

Psychiatric comorbidity related to obesity includes a range of mood, anxiety, substance use, somatoform, and eating disorders (EDs). In a study by Britz and colleagues[36] of obese adolescents seeking treatment of weight management, greater than 40% of the study population met Diagnostic and Statistical Manual of Mental Disorders, Fourth Edition (DSM-IV) criteria for a psychiatric illness. Elevated lifetime rates for mood (42.6%), anxiety (40.4%), substance use (36.2%), somatoform (14.9%), and EDs (17.0%) were reported compared with the general population. These elevated rates of psychopathology are similar to studies of adults, suggesting that mental health conditions presenting in childhood have augmenting effects on obesity.

Of the psychiatric conditions related to obesity, the most consistently reported association is that between depression and obesity. Weight gain, disordered eating, overweight, and obesity frequently occur in the context of mood disorders. Studies reflect the bidirectional relationship between obesity and depression without conclusive evidence of a causal relationship. Multiple factors, including iatrogenic causes such as psychotropic medications used to treat medical conditions, may induce mood symptoms.[37] Psychiatric illness and obesity have been established to be polygenic, heterogeneous conditions, impacted by factors such as family and social history, and environment. Prospective studies suggest that the onset of mood disorders may precede the development of overweight or obesity, perhaps in those individuals who are genetically predisposed.[38] It is important to note that most individuals who are obese or overweight do not have a mood disorder, but certain mood disorders, particularly atypical major depression, can be associated with weight gain and/or obesity.[38]

EDs have been specifically studied in relation to obesity, and the DSM-V changes in ED diagnoses aims to be more inclusive of the clinically relevant range of disordered eating. Weight preoccupation, binge eating, dieting, and purging are all weight-related problems that may co-occur or are behaviors that individuals transition between leading to EDs.[39] Recent research has demonstrated a significant association between the prevalence of EDs and weight status using criteria from the DSM-V. For example, prevalence of full or subthreshold bulimia nervosa increased from the normal-weight to the obese group, with an increased risk of 7.86 in men and 3.27 in women.[40] Contrary to what has been hypothesized and reported in adults,[41] binge eating disorder

(BED) is often associated with obesity, but no associations have been found between BED and particular BMI categories as of yet.[37,40]

COMBINED PREVENTION AND TREATMENT STRATEGIES

Continued investigations and discussions regarding the cause or consequence of obesity and mental health difficulties in children highlight the question of whether these problems are behavioral or psychiatric in origin. Although the origins of the combined health challenges may point to the provider type or treatment strategy best suited to manage the problem, another suggestion may be that these comorbid health difficulties are so interconnected and recalcitrant that a variety of treatment strategies is needed to effectively address both issues.

Approaches found to have the greatest impact in child overweight and obesity treatment include individual-level interventions that are multifaceted, which include motivational interviewing, effective problem-solving, and aspects of cognitive-behavior approaches.[8,33,42] The health effects of lifestyle modification approaches have been found to be sustained for longer periods of time,[43] and thus, it is recommended that overweight and obesity interventions with children emphasize a healthy lifestyle strategy over restrictive dieting or excessive physical activity. This approach places emphasis on health rather than weight or physical appearance.

Specific guidelines for treatment of childhood overweight and obesity have been outlined by the American Academy of Pediatrics[44] in which brief motivational interviewing strategies were included. Recommendations for a comprehensive review of systems include gaining information about psychiatric disorders (eg, anxiety, school avoidance, social isolation); this revision to the 1998 recommendations includes a significant focus on behavioral change strategies. Treatment interventions to improve child psychosocial health include a wide range of therapies, which are similar to the healthy lifestyle approach demonstrated to be effective with child obesity. These individualized treatment strategies often focus on a strengths-based approach such as promoting resilience and can be used as a treatment or a prevention strategy.

Multiple systematic reviews have been conducted with respect to child obesity in an effort to identify the most effective intervention elements.[45–52] Family involvement is frequently cited as a critical component to effective intervention. Similarly, approaches designed to enhance child psychosocial function and emotional wellness include family-focused intervention strategies. Although the need to include family seems essential and apparent when working with children, this represents a broader treatment strategy that shifts the perspective of addressing obesity and psychosocial wellness from an individual level concept to a more relational understanding of well-being embedded in a social-ecological framework. To date, limited intervention trials grounded by such a comprehensive framework have been conducted.[53–55]

A PARADIGM SHIFT FROM TREATMENT TO PREVENTION

Obesity is the result of people responding normally to the obesogenic environments they live in.[3] Environmental determinants of childhood obesity in the United States include modifications in food consumption, physical activity, screen time, and direct marketing of food to children.[56] Although implementation strategies exist for the adult population, prevention and early intervention strategies differ for children because the environment greatly influences children's food or activity choices. As a result, there is more opportunity for prevention efforts at a variety of different levels (ie, school, childcare, community, state and national policies). Behaviors that lead to obesity can be more easily modified in childhood and facilitated by environmental modifications (ie, safe areas for recreation, walking).

In an effort to accelerate the national progress to prevent and address childhood obesity, an Institute of Medicine committee published a set of recommendations in 2012.[57] This groundbreaking publication took a systems approach to the problem and outlined a comprehensive and integrated public health approach to preventing child obesity. The strategies outlined include health messaging and policy approaches in communities where children live and play. This community-based, whole-system approach to the obesity epidemic uses social change strategies and features 10 primary elements: (1) recognition of the public health problem, (2) capacity building around the health problem, (3) local creativity in intervention development, (4) strong relationships between organizations and with community, (5) wide-ranging and rich community engagement, (6) clear communications between community members and organizations, (7) embeddedness of action and policies for social/environmental change, (8) focus on robustness and sustainability of interventions, (9) facilitative leadership, and (10) articulated methods for outcome monitoring and evaluation. Such population-wide efforts are focused on strategies with a strong evidence base to achieve maximal impact in the environment and communities.

Single behavioral interventions, although effective strategies to improve individual wellness and reduce risk of comorbidities, are unlikely to have a substantial impact on the population health of our nation's children; therefore, a population focus is needed to address obesity.[58–60] There are several examples of effective community-based obesity prevention interventions with a public health focus that can be found in *Local Government Actions to Prevent Childhood Obesity* authored by the Institute of Medicine and National Research Council of the National Academies.[61] Identified studies include *Shape up Summerville* by Economos and colleagues[62,63]; *The Early Childhood Obesity Prevention Program (ECHO)* by Cloutier and colleagues[53]; and the *Health Eating and Active Communities Program (HEAC)*.[64,65] These and similar community-based, multilevel studies focus on evaluating the effects of multilevel approaches on the weight and health of child residents but do not consistently evaluate the intervention effects on the mental wellness of its child constituents.

The more conceptual and broad approaches to addressing child and adolescent obesity have been described in the literature (**Table 1**), each having their own strengths and limitations. High upfront costs have limited the universality of implementing prevention programs.[66] Sustained outcomes are an additional challenge particularly pertaining to obesity. However, when looking at prevention interventions for mental health, the converse is true. Although there are high upfront costs, the effects of interventions in mental health are often not recognized immediately, resulting in similar challenges of sustainability; stakeholders must recognize that effectiveness of interventions will only be realized in the long term and may be why there a paucity of research that includes public health approaches to promote child mental wellness.

An example of a public health prevention intervention with impact on both mental wellness and obesity would include breast-feeding. Breast-feeding has been shown to have health benefits for children at risk for childhood obesity.[67] In addition, child development and mental health are impacted as a result of breast-feeding, including higher IQ and promotion of attachment and bonding, again with longitudinal benefits.[68] Thus, national campaigns that encourage breast-feeding, programs that support the initiation of breast-feeding (ie, the Baby Friendly Hospital designation), and policy changes aimed to reduce social stigma that may dissuade mothers from breast-feeding (ie, elimination of national and state policies that forbid or restrict public

Table 1
Approach to prevention in child and adolescent obesity

Approach	Description	Examples	Strengths	Limitations
Clinical	Screening of at-risk individuals and applying evidence-based treatment intervention to reduce burden of disease	Identification of children with BMI percentiles in the overweight/obese range to provide targeted intervention	Application of evidence-based treatment for a target population	High-cost, time-limited benefit (except for bariatric surgery)
Public health	Health promotion strategies	School-based health programs; implementation of policies protecting children from direct food marketing	Prevention-based, minimizing number of children developing obesity	High upfront cost with long-term benefits, which are not immediately seen and may have varied results
"Free" market	Individual choices are emphasized with limited governmental intervention based on a well-informed consumer	Market shifts to provide better options based on parent/child demand for healthier choices	Individuals satisfy their own preferences	Overconsumption profits are too great and drive the overall economy
Human rights	Based on the Convention of the Rights of a Child (World Health Organization) for basic rights to adequate food and health; society is responsible to provide these to children	Societies assume responsibility to provide a healthy environment and food to children	Obesity would be greatly reduced if this was universally accepted	Ideal framework but implementation is challenging at the societal level
Risks/benefits	Balance the health risks associated with the economic profitability of promoting high-energy foods and sedentary lifestyle	Profit margins on obesogenic products are limited due to marketing restrictions based on known risks in promoting obesity	Increased transparency with risk analysis of consumer marketing impacting obesity	Controversial outcomes; least effective strategy to minimize childhood obesity as they have limited means to make changes to the market

Data from Swinburn B. Obesity prevention in children and adolescents. Child Adolesc Psychiatric Clin 2008;18(1):209–23.

breast-feeding) have been found to be an important element of a comprehensive approach to addressing child obesity and mental wellness.

There are several psychosocial factors contributing to the obesity epidemic. It is reported that today's children are engaged in screen time activities an average of 7 hours a day.[69] The American Academy of Pediatrics recommends that screen time be limited to 2 hours per day. Without addressing media content, the overall lack of physical activity and sensory stimulation related to excess screen time has been shown to lead to attention problems, school difficulties, sleep disorders, EDs, and obesity.[70] The advertisements of unhealthy dietary options that proliferate TV programming and target children and adolescent viewers additionally should be targeted as a public health issue.

The pressing need to decrease screen time for children and adolescents is being addressed in multiple ways. Many afterschool care organizations and childcare organizations have enacted rules that limit the use and availability of screen time for the children in their care. In addition, many organizations are increasing and/or strengthening the type and number of non-screen-time activities and programs available for all children to participate in. In some instances, unique funding sources have been sought (ie, angel donor programs, insurance company support) to make safe supervised recreational activities available for children at high risk for obesity. Increasing the availability of safe, adult-supervised, physical and recreational activities impacts the mental wellness of children as well.

Evidence on the mental health benefits of exercise in children and adolescents is increasing. A study by Pontifex and colleagues[71] assessed the effect of exercise in children with attention deficit hyperactivity disorder. In this study, children 8 to 10 years of age showed greater accuracy on attention control tasks and academic performance. Studies looking at the impact of exercise on adolescent depression have noted that youth who engage in 60 minutes of physical activity per day are less likely to have depressive symptoms.[72] There is a growing body of evidence regarding the long-term benefits of children engaged in physical and recreational activities. Multilevel intervention strategies need to be supported and promoted by the systems surrounding children because their influence helps to provide safe environments and allows youth to explore active opportunities.

SUMMARY AND DISCUSSION: THE FUTURE OF CHILD MENTAL AND PHYSICAL HEALTH RESEARCH AND PRACTICE EFFORTS
Epigenetic Influences

Not only the scope and level of intervention strategies should be considered when addressing obesity and mental wellness, but also understanding the generational impact of this dyadic health challenge is a focus of some contemporary investigations. Just as genetic and familial linkages have been implicated with regard to obesity and mental health issues,[73–75] the relationships between potential epigenetic changes, toxic stress, and allostatic load as a result of obesity, chronic inflammation, chronic stress, and comorbid psychosocial challenges within and across generations are being explored.[76–79]

The overlap of epigenetic factors contributing to both obesity and mental disorders (ie, chronic toxic stress) is pronounced, and prevention strategies for either can have dual influence. Looking at these common epigenetic factors, parallels are sought to implement single strategic interventions using a socioecological approach (**Table 2**). For child health, these efforts have a common root starting in infancy, and promotion of health should be emphasized rather than dichotomizing physical and mental health. Examples of factors that contribute to these successes include prenatal care, healthy

Table 2
Parallels in the socioecological approach to prevention in childhood obesity and mental health disorders in consideration of common epigenetic influences

Socioecological Aspect	Obesity	Influences	Mental Health
Individual	• Encourage behavioral activation • Promote healthy lifestyle decision-making over appearance focus • Include problem-solving	• Gender • Physical activity • Self-esteem • Emotional/cognitive maturity • Physical health	• Promotion of resilience • Enhance individual skills • Encourage academic achievement • Assessment of genetic risk factors • Minimize/avoid substance use
Family	• Provide parenting coaching/education about health • Encourage health promotion/prevention for families • Encourage role modeling healthy behaviors • Establish clear boundaries regarding family eating and screen time rules	• Breast-feeding • Attachment/bonding • Maternal depression • Caregiver education • Abuse/neglect • Economic security • Family physical or mental illness	• Address caregiver wellness • Promote family strengths • Implement evidence-based parenting programs • Use home visiting programs to improve pregnancy outcomes and reduce abuse and neglect
Community	• Advocate for school nutritional and physical activity programs • Provide safe environments to promote outdoor activity • Discourage weight-based victimization and bullying	• Exposure to violence • Access to health care • School environment • Public safety • Access to health-promoting activities	• Provide safe environment to decrease community violence • Implement policies for school bullying/peer victimization • Increase school mental health services • Increase equitable access to health care
Societal	• Implement restrictions on direct marketing to children • Strengthen healthy nutrition policies • Enhance and encourage built environment initiatives • Discourage political barriers to health promoting behaviors • Strengthen health-promoting food and beverage retailing and distribution policies • Support federal programs that support healthy nutrition	• Policy/legislation • Adherence to health standards • Stigma • Discrimination • Allocation of resources • Research-driven initiatives	• Advocate for equal access to various levels of mental health care • Minimize societal stigma through public education • Allocate resources for childhood mental health prevention • Implement standards for mental health support for children in foster care • Establish parity between medical and mental health needs

Adapted from National Research Council (US), Institute of Medicine (US) Committee on the Prevention of Mental Disorders and Substance Abuse Among Children, Youth, and Young Adults: Research Advances and Promising Interventions, O'Connell ME, Boat T, editors. Preventing mental, emotional, and behavioral disorder among young people: progress and possibilities. Washington DC: National Academies Press; 2009.

birth weight, breast-feeding, positive parent management training, home visitation, school interventions, universal screening, routine well child visits to primary care, and anticipatory guidance.[80] These factors are specific examples of the basic elements of health care that include prevention, acute care, and chronic care management.[81]

Combined Mental and Physical Health Implementation Investigations

As described herein, there is a large and continuously growing foundation of rigorously conducted research that provides the evidence to guide clinical practice regarding the treatment and prevention of obesity and comorbid psychosocial problems. Rigorous research is characterized by a high level of controlled conditions that do not generalize into real-world settings and may result in variable health outcomes in the general population. In addition, there is limited research addressing both aspects of health that has been conducted within community settings, the places where children and families live, work, and play. However, intervention at a community level is more likely to impact the many issues that cause the tightly interconnected coexistence of childhood obesity and psychosocial morbidity.

Implementation research with communities of individuals at high risk is needed to test these recalcitrant health threats. Given the interconnectedness of psychosocial impairments, psychiatric conditions, and obesity in children, a public health approach to preventing and addressing the predictors, comorbidities, and/or sequelae of child obesity with a focus on health and wellness may be an important strategy to embrace. Most effective and innovative strategies to address obesity prevention would require the participation of interprofessional teams of policymakers, health care providers, and organizations that provide care, education, and supervision of children, teens, and families (ie, schools, childcare centers, community centers).

REFERENCES

1. Ogden CL, Carroll MD, Kit BK, et al. Prevalence of childhood and adult obesity in the United States, 2011-2012. JAMA 2014;311(8):806–14.
2. Mitchell NS, Catenacci VA, Wyatt HR, et al. Obesity: overview of an epidemic. Psychiatr Clin North Am 2011;34(4):717–32.
3. Swinburn BA, Sacks G, Hall KD, et al. The global obesity pandemic: shaped by global drivers and local environments. Lancet 2011;378(9793):804–14.
4. Melnyk BM, Small L, Moore N. The worldwide epidemic of child and adolescent overweight and obesity: calling all clinicians and researchers to intensify efforts in prevention and treatment. Worldviews Evid Based Nurs 2008;5(3):109–12.
5. Sahoo K, Sahoo B, Choudhury AK, et al. Childhood obesity: causes and consequences. J Family Med Prim Care 2015;4(2):187–92.
6. Pulgaron ER. Childhood obesity: a review of increased risk for physical and psychological comorbidities. Clin Ther 2013;35(1):A18–32.
7. Harriger JA, Thompson JK. Psychological consequences of obesity: weight bias and body image in overweight and obese youth. Int Rev Psychiatry 2012;24(3):247–53.
8. Zametkin AJ, Zoon CK, Klein HW, et al. Psychiatric aspects of child and adolescent obesity: a review of the past 10 years. J Am Acad Child Adolesc Psychiatry 2004;43(2):134–50.
9. Vander Wal JS, Mitchell ER. Psychological complications of pediatric obesity. Pediatr Clin North Am 2011;58(6):1393–401, x.

10. Cornette R. The emotional impact of obesity on children. Worldviews Evid Based Nurs 2008;5(3):136–41.
11. Epstein LH, Paluch RA, Gordy CC, et al. Decreasing sedentary behaviors in treating pediatric obesity. Arch Pediatr Adolesc Med 2000;154(3):220–6.
12. Barlow SE, Trowbridge FL, Klish WJ, et al. Treatment of child and adolescent obesity: reports from pediatricians, pediatric nurse practitioners, and registered dieticians. Pediatrics 2002;110(1):229–35.
13. Incledon E, Wake M, Hay M. Psychological predictors of adiposity: systematic review of longitudinal studies. Int J Pediatr Obes 2011;6(2–2):e1–11.
14. White B, Nicholls D, Christie D, et al. Childhood psychological function and obesity risk across the lifecourse: findings from the 1970 British Cohort Study. Int J Obes (Lond) 2012;36(4):511–6.
15. Goodwin RD, Sourander A, Duarte CS, et al. Do mental health problems in childhood predict chronic physical conditions among males in early adulthood? Evidence from a community-based prospective study. Psychol Med 2009;39(2):301–11.
16. Chang Y, Gable S. Predicting weight status stability and change from fifth grade to eighth grade: the significant role of adolescents' social-emotional well-being. J Adolesc Health 2013;52(4):448–55.
17. Geoffroy MC, Li L, Power C. Depressive symptoms and body mass index: co-morbidity and direction of association in a British birth cohort followed over 50 years. Psychol Med 2014;44(12):2641–52.
18. Larsen JK, Otten R, Fisher JO, et al. Depressive symptoms in adolescence: a poor indicator of increases in body mass index. J Adolesc Health 2014;54(1):94–9.
19. Datar A, Sturm R. Childhood overweight and parent- and teacher-reported behavior problems: evidence from a prospective study of kindergartners. Arch Pediatr Adolesc Med 2004;158(8):804–10.
20. Wang F, Wild TC, Kipp W, et al. The influence of childhood obesity on the development of self-esteem. Health Rep 2009;20(2):21–7.
21. Gable S, Krull JL, Chang Y. Boys' and girls' weight status and math performance from kindergarten entry through fifth grade: a mediated analysis. Child Dev 2012;83(5):1822–39.
22. Cui W, Zack MM, Wethington H. Health-related quality of life and body mass index among US adolescents. Qual Life Res 2014;23(7):2139–50.
23. Taylor VH, Forhan M, Vigod SN, et al. The impact of obesity on quality of life. Best Pract Res Clin Endocrinol Metab 2013;27(2):139–46.
24. Morrison KM, Shin S, Tarnopolsky M, et al. Association of depression & health related quality of life with body composition in children and youth with obesity. J Affect Disord 2014;172C:18–23.
25. Wu YP, Steele RG. Predicting health-related quality of life from the psychosocial profiles of youth seeking treatment for obesity. J Dev Behav Pediatr 2013;34(8):575–82.
26. Williams JW, Canterford L, Hesketh KD, et al. Changes in body mass index and health related quality of life from childhood to adolescence. Int J Pediatr Obes 2011;6(2–2):e442–8.
27. Bryan AD, Fisher JD, Fisher WA, et al. Understanding condom use among heroin addicts in methadone maintenance using the information-motivation-behavioral skills model. Subst Use Misuse 2000;35(4):451–71.
28. Griffiths LJ, Wolke D, Page AS, et al, ALSPAC Study Team. Obesity and bullying: different effects for boys and girls. Arch Dis Child 2006;91(2):121–5.

29. Johnson NB, Hayes LD, Brown K, et al, Centers for Disease Control and Prevention (CDC). CDC National Health Report: leading causes of morbidity and mortality and associated behavioral risk and protective factors–United States, 2005-2013. MMWR Surveill Summ 2014;63(Suppl 4):3–27.
30. Huang DY, Lanza HI, Wright-Volel K, et al. Developmental trajectories of childhood obesity and risk behaviors in adolescence. J Adolesc 2013;36(1): 139–48.
31. Ratcliff MB, Jenkins TM, Reiter-Purtill J, et al. Risk-taking behaviors of adolescents with extreme obesity: normative or not? Pediatrics 2011;127(5):827–34.
32. Zeller MH, Reiter-Purtill J, Jenkins TM, et al. Adolescent suicidal behavior across the excess weight status spectrum. Obesity (Silver Spring) 2013;21(5):1039–45.
33. Scheimann AO. Overview of pediatric obesity for the pediatric mental health provider. Int Rev Psychiatry 2012;24(3):231–40.
34. Kovacs M, Goldston D, Obrosky DS, et al. Prevalence and predictors of pervasive noncompliance with medical treatment among youths with insulin-dependent diabetes mellitus. J Am Acad Child Adolesc Psychiatry 1992;31(6): 1112–9.
35. Janicke DM, Harman JS, Kelleher KJ, et al. Psychiatric diagnosis in children and adolescents with obesity-related health conditions. J Dev Behav Pediatr 2008; 29(4):276–84.
36. Britz B, Siegfried W, Ziegler A, et al. Rates of psychiatric disorders in a clinical study group of adolescents with extreme obesity and in obese adolescents ascertained via a population based study. Int J Obes Relat Metab Disord 2000; 24(12):1707–14.
37. Kjelsas E, Bjornstrom C, Gotestam KG. Prevalence of eating disorders in female and male adolescents (14-15 years). Eat Behav 2004;5(1):13–25.
38. McElroy SL, Kotwal R, Malhotra S, et al. Are mood disorders and obesity related? A review for the mental health professional. J Clin Psychiatry 2004;65(5):634–51 [quiz: 730].
39. Neumark-Sztainer DR, Wall MM, Haines JI, et al. Shared risk and protective factors for overweight and disordered eating in adolescents. Am J Prev Med 2007; 33(5):359–69.
40. Flament MF, Henderson K, Buchholz A, et al. Weight status and DSM-5 diagnoses of eating disorders in adolescents from the community. J Am Acad Child Adolesc Psychiatry 2015;54(5):403–11.e2.
41. Hudson JI, Hiripi E, Pope HG Jr, et al. The prevalence and correlates of eating disorders in the national comorbidity survey replication. Biol Psychiatry 2007; 61(3):348–58.
42. Wilfley DE, Kass AE, Kolko RP. Counseling and behavior change in pediatric obesity. Pediatr Clin North Am 2011;58(6):1403–24, x.
43. Martin A, Saunders DH, Shenkin SD, et al. Lifestyle intervention for improving school achievement in overweight or obese children and adolescents. Cochrane Database Syst Rev 2014;(3):CD009728.
44. American Academy of Pediatrics. Prevention of pediatric overweight and obesity. Pediatrics 2003;112(424):430.
45. Redsell SA, Edmonds B, Swift JA, et al. Systematic review of randomized controlled trials of interventions that aim to reduce the risk, either directly or indirectly, of overweight and obesity in infancy and early childhood. Matern Child Nutr 2015. http://dx.doi.org/10.1111/mcn.12184.
46. Wang Y, Cai L, Wu Y, et al. What childhood obesity prevention programs work? A systematic review and meta-analysis. Obes Rev 2015;16(7):547–65.

47. Kelishadi R, Azizi-Soleiman F. Controlling childhood obesity: a systematic review on strategies and challenges. J Res Med Sci 2014;19(10):993–1008.
48. Cai L, Wu Y, Cheskin LJ, et al. Effect of childhood obesity prevention programs on blood lipids: a systematic review and meta-analysis. Obes Rev 2014;15(12):933–44.
49. Avery A, Bostock L, McCullough F. A systematic review investigating interventions that can help reduce consumption of sugar-sweetened beverages in children leading to changes in body fatness. J Hum Nutr Diet 2015;28(Suppl 1):52–64.
50. Barr-Anderson DJ, Singleton C, Cotwright CJ, et al. Outside-of-school time obesity prevention and treatment interventions in African American youth. Obes Rev 2014;15(Suppl 4):26–45.
51. Laws R, Campbell KJ, van der Pligt P, et al. The impact of interventions to prevent obesity or improve obesity related behaviours in children (0-5 years) from socio-economically disadvantaged and/or indigenous families: a systematic review. BMC Public Health 2014;14:779.
52. Temple M, Robinson JC. A systematic review of interventions to promote physical activity in the preschool setting. J Spec Pediatr Nurs 2014;19(4):274–84.
53. Cloutier MM, Wiley J, Wang Z, et al. The early childhood obesity prevention program (ECHO): an ecologically-based intervention delivered by home visitors for newborns and their mothers. BMC Public Health 2015;15:584.
54. Lytle LA. Dealing with the childhood obesity epidemic: a public health approach. Abdom Imaging 2012;37(5):719–24.
55. Yancey AK, Kumanyika SK, Ponce NA, et al. Population-based interventions engaging communities of color in healthy eating and active living: a review. Prev Chronic Dis 2004;1(1):A09.
56. Centers for Disease Control and Prevention (CDC). CDC grand rounds: childhood obesity in the United States. MMWR Morb Mortal Wkly Rep 2011;60(2):42–6.
57. Institute of Medicine of the National Academies. Committee on accelerating progress in obesity prevention, food and nutrition board. In: Glickman D, Parker L, Sim LJ, et al, editors. Washington, DC: Institute of Medicine; 2012.
58. Wang SS, Brownell KD. Public policy and obesity: the need to marry science with advocacy. Psychiatr Clin North Am 2005;28(1):235–52, x.
59. Novak NL, Brownell KD. Role of policy and government in the obesity epidemic. Circulation 2012;126(19):2345–52.
60. Novak NL, Brownell KD. Obesity: a public health approach. Psychiatr Clin North Am 2011;34(4):895–909.
61. Sanchez E, Burns AC, Parker L. Local government actions to prevent childhood obesity. Washington, DC: National Academies Press; 2009.
62. Economos CD, Hyatt RR, Must A, et al. Shape Up Somerville two-year results: a community-based environmental change intervention sustains weight reduction in children. Prev Med 2013;57(4):322–7.
63. Economos CD, Hyatt RR, Goldberg JP, et al. A community intervention reduces BMI z-score in children: shape up somerville first year results. Obesity (Silver Spring) 2007;15(5):1325–36.
64. Cheadle A, Samuels SE, Rauzon S, et al. Approaches to measuring the extent and impact of environmental change in three California community-level obesity prevention initiatives. Am J Public Health 2010;100(11):2129–36.
65. Samuels SE, Craypo L, Boyle M, et al. The California endowment's healthy eating, active communities program: a midpoint review. Am J Public Health 2010;100(11):2114–23.

66. National Research Council (US), Institute of Medicine (US) Committee on the Prevention of Mental Disorders and Substance Abuse Among Children, Youth, and Young Adults: Research Advances and Promising Interventions, O'Connell ME, Boat T, editors. Preventing mental, emotional, and behavioral disorder among young people: progress and possibilities. Washington, DC: National Academies Press; 2009. doi: NBK32775. [book accession].

67. Harder T, Bergmann R, Kallischnigg G, et al. Duration of breastfeeding and risk of overweight: a meta-analysis. Am J Epidemiol 2005;162(5):397–403.

68. Horta BL, de Mola CL, Victora CG. Breastfeeding and intelligence: systematic review and meta-analysis. Acta Paediatr 2015;104(467):14–9.

69. Hinkley T, Salmon J, Okely AD, et al. Preschoolers' physical activity, screen time, and compliance with recommendations. Med Sci Sports Exerc 2012;44(3): 458–65.

70. Foster E, O'Keeffe M, Matthews JN, et al. Children's estimates of food portion size: the effect of timing of dietary interview on the accuracy of children's portion size estimates. Br J Nutr 2008;99(1):185–90.

71. Pontifex MB, Saliba BJ, Raine LB, et al. Exercise improves behavioral, neurocognitive, and scholastic performance in children with attention-deficit/hyperactivity disorder. J Pediatr 2013;162(3):543–51.

72. Kremer P, Elshaug C, Leslie E, et al. Physical activity, leisure-time screen use and depression among children and young adolescents. J Sci Med Sport 2014;17(2): 183–7.

73. Micali N, Field AE, Treasure JL, et al. Are obesity risk genes associated with binge eating in adolescence? Obesity (Silver Spring) 2015;23(8):1729–36.

74. Porfirio MC, Giovinazzo S, Cortese S, et al. Role of ADHD symptoms as a contributing factor to obesity in patients with MC4R mutations. Med Hypotheses 2015; 84(1):4–7.

75. Scott S. Parenting quality and children's mental health: biological mechanisms and psychological interventions. Curr Opin Psychiatry 2012;25(4):301–6.

76. Padilla MA, Elobeid M, Ruden DM, et al. An examination of the association of selected toxic metals with total and central obesity indices: NHANES 99-02. Int J Environ Res Public Health 2010;7(9):3332–47.

77. Sinha R, Jastreboff AM. Stress as a common risk factor for obesity and addiction. Biol Psychiatry 2013;73(9):827–35.

78. Katz DA, Sprang G, Cooke C. The cost of chronic stress in childhood: understanding and applying the concept of allostatic load. Psychodyn Psychiatry 2012;40(3):469–80.

79. Barkin S, Rao Y, Smith P, et al. A novel approach to the study of pediatric obesity: a biomarker model. Pediatr Ann 2012;41(6):250–6.

80. Quante M, Hesse M, Dohnert M, et al. The LIFE child study: a life course approach to disease and health. BMC Public Health 2012;12:1021.

81. Arora S, Kalishman S, Dion D, et al. Partnering urban academic medical centers and rural primary care clinicians to provide complex chronic disease care. Health Aff (Millwood) 2011;30(6):1176–84.

Human Immunodeficiency Virus Prevention

 CrossMark

Teaniese Latham Davis, PhD, MPH[a],*, Ralph DiClemente, PhD[b]

KEYWORDS

- HIV • AIDS • Prevention • Behavioral intervention • Biomedical intervention
- Treatment • Medication adherence

KEY POINTS

- Human immunodeficiency virus (HIV) transmission can be prevented through reducing sexual risk and needle/equipment sharing.
- Primary and secondary prevention are essential to reducing HIV incidence and prevalence.
- Evidence-based interventions are classified into 3 categories: behavioral interventions, biomedical interventions, and linkage to, retention in, and re-engagement in HIV care.

INTRODUCTION

Human immunodeficiency virus (HIV) is the virus that causes AIDS. Surveillance data from 2012 indicate an estimated 1.2 million people aged 13 years and older were living with HIV infection in the United States, of whom 12.8% do not know their status. According to estimates from the Centers for Disease Control and Prevention (CDC), there are approximately 50,000 new HIV infections annually.[1]

Human Immunodeficiency Virus Disparities

Estimates from 2010 data on new HIV infections among subpopulations indicate the highest number of new HIV infections occurred among white men who have sex with men (MSM), followed by black and Hispanic/Latino MSM, accounting for approximately 72% of all new HIV infections in 2010.[2,3] Racial disparities exist in the rate of new HIV infections. Although black Americans accounted for 12% of the US population, they accounted for 44% of all new HIV infections in 2010. Black women represented 29% of all new HIV infections in 2010, a 21% decrease since 2008.[2]

Drs T.L. Davis and R. DiClemente do not have any commercial or financial conflicts of interest and any funding sources to disclose.

[a] Public Health Sciences Institute, Morehouse College, 830 Westview Drive Southwest, Atlanta, GA 30314, USA; [b] Department of Behavioral Sciences and Health Education, Rollins School of Public Health, Emory University, 1518 Clifton Road Northeast, Atlanta, GA 30322, USA

* Corresponding author.

E-mail address: teaniese.davis@morehouse.edu

There are 4 modes of HIV transmission:

1. Sexual behavior
2. Sharing needles
3. Blood transfusions
4. Mother-to-child via pregnancy, childbirth, or breastfeeding

Human Immunodeficiency Virus Transmission

HIV in the United States is most commonly spread through oral, anal, or vaginal sex with a partner who is HIV positive or by sharing needles, or other equipment used to inject drugs, with someone who is HIV positive. Anal sex has the highest risk disease transmission, followed by vaginal sex, with receptive anal sex being riskier than insertive anal sex. Having multiple sexually transmitted infections (STIs), multiple sex partners, and nonmonogamous (concurrent) sex partners increases the risk for sexual transmission of HIV. Other less common modes of transmission in the United States include blood transfusions and perinatal transmission from HIV-positive pregnant mother to her child during pregnancy, birth, or breastfeeding. Although oral sex is less risky than anal and vaginal sex, giving fellatio (mouth to penis) and having a partner ejaculate semen into the partner's mouth are riskier oral sex behaviors.[4]

Human Immunodeficiency Virus Prevention

With no available cure for HIV, primary prevention to reduce incident cases of HIV is essential. The following strategies reduce HIV transmission[5]:

- Abstinence from oral, anal, and vaginal sex
- Engage in less risky sexual behaviors
- Correctly and consistently use condoms and latex barriers (such as dental dams) during oral, anal, and vaginal sex
- Limit the number of sex partners
- Get tested for HIV and other STIs and have sex partners engage in routine testing; the CDC recommends annual testing for sexually active individuals.
- Pre-exposure prophylaxis (PrEP) is a doctor-prescribed medication taken daily to prevent HIV infection; PrEP is recommended for HIV-negative individuals in a high-risk sexual relationship, which includes having a sex partner who is HIV positive.
- Postexposure prophylaxis is a doctor-prescribed medication that reduces the risk of HIV transmission for HIV-negative individuals who have possibly been exposed to HIV.

Primary prevention reduces transmission of HIV, ensuring fewer people become infected from individuals who are HIV positive. Secondary prevention is a key factor to prevent being infected with a new strain of HIV or infecting another person. Secondary prevention also reduces the severity of HIV by early identification of cases through testing and rapid intervention.[6]

Human Immunodeficiency Virus Risk Factors

In addition to encouraging safer sexual behaviors to prevent HIV transmission, research has examined the role of substance use and mental illness related to an increased risk for HIV infection. Among Medicaid beneficiaries with mental illness, reporting substance abuse/dependence was significantly predictive of new HIV diagnoses. However, in the absence of alcohol use, a serious mental illness (SMI) diagnosis was not associated with an increased risk of HIV acquisition.[7]

To understand the pathway in which a mental illness diagnosis leads to an increased risk in HIV and other STIs, research has examined the association between mental illness and sexual risk behaviors. Among a sample of black adolescents, having depressive symptoms was associated with using condoms less frequently compared with their counterparts without depressive symptoms.[8]

In addition to risky sexual behaviors, there is also an association between mental illness and drug use, another risk behavior for HIV acquisition.[9] Research indicates that women experiencing mental illness have significantly higher drug use. Furthermore, in a sample of incarcerated women, those with posttraumatic stress disorder (PTSD) and depression were more likely to engage in injection drug use (IDU), a risk behavior for HIV acquisition, compared with nonincarcerated women without PTSD.[10] Research indicated a similar association between PTSD and sexual risk behavior among younger gay men (aged 20–29 years); the same association did not hold true for older gay men (aged 30+ years).[11]

The prevalence of mental illness can range among different subsamples of the US population. Among incarcerated women, the prevalence of mental illness was 80% in one study.[10] Among gay/bisexual men, a subgroup with the high HIV infection rates, 47% of men met the criteria for at least one anxiety disorder; 14% met the criteria for at least 2 anxiety disorders, and 3.5% met the criteria for at least 3 anxiety disorders.[11]

Treatment for People Living with Human Immunodeficiency Virus

Doctors prescribe antiretroviral therapy (ART) for people living with HIV to suppress the HIV viral load present in their bodies. Keeping the viral load low does the following[12]:

- Reduces the risk for HIV transmission to others
- Increases the likelihood of a normal life expectancy for people living with HIV

For HIV-positive individuals, nonadherence to HIV medication can result in increased viral loads. To keep viral load levels undetectable, research indicates that individuals must have almost perfect adherence to the medication regimen prescribed.[13] Nonadherence to medication can lead to drug-resistant HIV variants that can result in treatment failure.[14]

As of 2011, CDC estimates, using national surveillance data, indicated that 1.2 million people were living with HIV in the United States, of whom:

- 86% were diagnosed with HIV
- 40% were linked to medical care
- 37% were prescribed ART
- 30% reached viral suppression

A key factor in increasing the percentage of HIV-positive individuals who have a suppressed viral load is to (1) increase testing to reduce the number of undiagnosed HIV infections, which is currently approximately 20%; and (2) increase the percentage of people living with HIV who are linked to and engaged in medical care.[12]

Challenges to Human Immunodeficiency Virus Medication Adherence

There are multiple barriers that decrease medication adherence among people living with HIV,[15] as listed[16]:

- SMI
- Substance abuse

- Homelessness
- Low education and literacy levels
- High pill burden (ie, medication requiring a particular food regimen, multiple side effects, multiple doses required daily)
- Characteristics of the clinical setting (settings that are not comprehensive)

Considering these barriers, factors that enhance HIV medication adherence include the following:

- Comprehensive clinical setting, providing care to support complex needs of patients, involving care from pharmacists, social workers, case managers, psychiatrists
- Patient-provider relationship with open communication and in a nonjudgmental environment

The prevalence of HIV among people with mental illness is higher than the prevalence of HIV among people in the general population. In addition to the disproportionate prevalence of HIV among people with SMI, comorbid HIV and SMI increase health care costs.[17] People living with SMI and HIV are more likely to have poor adherence to HIV medication.[18]

INTERVENTIONS
Behavioral Interventions

Effective behavioral interventions to reduce the risk of HIV transmission focus on teaching correct condom skills, negotiating condom use using effective communication, and encouraging individual and partner testing. These interventions have resulted in reductions in incident STI infections, increased condom use, and reductions in sex partners.[19] CDC refers to these as high-impact interventions (HIP). There are 84 behavioral interventions available through the CDCs' Effective Interventions Web site. These interventions are packaged and include the materials necessary for implementation.[20]

Biomedical Interventions

Biomedical interventions focus on preventing HIV infection, reducing susceptibility to HIV, and decreasing HIV infectiousness using public health strategies. Among people living with HIV, ART is an effective public health strategy to reduce the risk for HIV transmission and improve health outcomes. Effective and comprehensive prevention efforts include (1) finding individuals who are infected with HIV, (2) providing linkages to and retaining them in care, and (3) assisting with medication adherence to suppress their viral load. This coordinated care is essential.

There are 10 medication adherence evidence-based interventions available through the CDC's Effective Interventions site and 9 Best Practices for promoting linkage to care and retention in HIV care.[20] To assist with medication adherence, CDC has an e-Learning Training Toolkit for medical providers called Every Dose Every Day. The tool kit includes 4 evidence-based strategies[21]:

1. HEART (Helping Enhance Adherence to Antiretroviral Therapy): An intervention administered before and during the first 2 months after people begin ART. HEART involves providing social support and problem-solving skills and works with people living with HIV to identify a support partner.
2. SMART (Sharing Medical Adherence Responsibilities Together) Couples: An intervention for serodiscordant couples whereby one person is HIV negative and one

person is HIV positive. SMART Couples includes ART medication adherence and sexual risk reduction strategies for couples.

3. Peer Support: An intervention focused on having people who are HIV positive and adherent to ART offers support to peers related to medication adherence.

4. Partnership for Health for Medication adherence: A provider-administered and clinic-based individual-level intervention focused on enhancing the patient-provider relationship to promote medication adherence for HIV-positive patients.

Other biomedical interventions[22] include courses to support medication adherence targeting physicians and other health care providers:

1. The Prevention Benefit of ART for HIV-infected Patients: A Web-based course for physicians focused on prevention benefits of ART. This course qualifies for 125 units of continuing medical education and is free of charge.

2. Prevention with [HIV] Positives (PwP) in Action: A 30-minute graphic novel to serve as an example of a collaborative strategy to implement PwP.

Table 1 presents a list of biomedical and behavioral HIV interventions and indicates the risk category and intervention type.

Linkage to, Retention in, and Re-Engagement in Human Immunodeficiency Virus Care Interventions

Given the importance of connecting people to care who are living with HIV or AIDS, known as the care continuum, it is essential to have interventions with evidence of efficacy or effectiveness.[19] In a review of interventions to promote linkage to care, multiple interventions increased the percentage of people entering care who were newly diagnosed with HIV, with 78% to 92% of study participants entering the care continuum within 3 to 6 months of receiving the intervention.[23] Effective strategies for engaging patients in the care continuum[23] include case managers assisting clients navigate the care continuum by

- Providing psychological support and counseling
- Building a relationship with patients
- Providing information and education
- Identifying client needs and strengths
- Attending appointments with clients
- Coordinating appointments for clients
- Providing transportation, housing, clothing, food resources
- Encouraging patient/provider communication
- Addressing stigma
- Supplying referrals to substance abuse treatment and harm reduction equipment

There are 11 linkage to, retention in, and re-engagement in HIV care best practices for HIV-positive patients, of which 5 are evidence-based interventions and 6 are evidence-informed interventions.[19]

Structural Interventions

These interventions are designed to effect change on a policy, societal, or organizational level. Examples of structural interventions include condom distribution programs (CDP) and needle distribution and exchange programs.[24]

Condom distribution

CDPs increase access to condoms to increase safer sex strategies and reduce the likelihood of HIV transmission. Research indicates CDPs prevent HIV infections, are

Table 1
Behavioral and biomedical interventions for primary and secondary Human Immunodeficiency Virus prevention

Intervention Name	Intervention Type		Risk Category				
	Medication Adherence	Behavioral Risk Reduction	Drug Users	Heterosexual Adults	High-Risk Youth	MSM	People Living with HIV/AIDS
Adapted Stage Enhanced Motivational Interviewing (A-SEMI)	—	×	—	×	—	—	—
Amigas	—	×	—	×	—	—	—
Assisting in Rehabilitating Kids (ARK)	—	×	—	—	×	—	—
Becoming a Responsible Teen (BART)	—	×	—	—	×	—	—
Be Proud! Be Responsible!	—	×	—	—	×	—	—
Brief Alcohol Intervention for Needle Exchange (BRAINE)	—	×	×	—	—	—	—
Brief Group Counseling	—	×	—	—	—	×	—
CARE+	×	×	—	—	—	×	×
Centering Pregnancy Plus (CPP)	—	×	—	×	—	—	—
Chat	—	×	—	×	—	—	—
Choices	—	×	—	×	—	—	—
Choosing Life: Empowerment, Action Results (CLEAR)	—	×	×	×	—	×	×
Cognitive Behavioral STD/HIV Prevention (CE-AP)	—	×	—	×	—	—	—
Community Promise	—	×	×	×	—	×	—
Condom Promotion	—	×	—	×	—	—	—
Connect	—	×	—	×	—	—	—
Connect 2	—	×	—	×	—	—	—
Directly Administered Antiretroviral Therapy (DAART)	×	—	×	—	—	—	—

	1	2	3	4	5	6	7
Doing Something Different	—	×	—	×	—	—	—
Drug Users Intervention Trial (DUIT)	—	×	×	—	—	—	—
Eban	—	×	×	×	—	—	×
EXPLORE	—	×	—	—	—	×	—
Familias Unidas	—	×	—	—	×	—	—
Female and Culturally Specific Negotiation	—	×	×	×	—	—	—
Female Condom Skills Training	—	×	—	×	—	—	—
FIO: The Future Is Ours	—	×	—	×	—	—	—
Focus on Youth	—	×	—	—	×	—	—
Focus on Youth + ImPACT	—	×	—	—	×	—	—
FOF: Focus on Future	—	×	—	×	—	—	—
Health Improvement Project (HIP)	—	×	—	×	—	—	×
HIP Teens	—	×	—	—	×	—	—
Healthy Living Project (HLP)	×	×	—	—	—	×	—
Healthy Love	—	×	—	×	—	—	—
Healthy Relationships	—	×	—	—	—	×	×
HIV Education and Testing	—	×	—	×	—	—	—
HoMBReS	—	×	—	×	—	—	—
HORIZONS	—	×	—	—	×	—	—
¡Cuídate!	—	×	—	—	×	—	—
In the Mix	×	×	—	×	—	—	×
Insights	—	×	—	×	—	—	—
Intensive AIDS Education	—	×	×	—	×	—	—
"Light"	—	×	—	×	—	—	—
Living in the Face of Trauma (LIFT)	—	×	—	—	—	—	×
MAALES	—	×	—	—	—	×	—

(continued on next page)

Table 1
(continued)

Intervention Name	Intervention Type		Risk Category				
	Medication Adherence	Behavioral Risk Reduction	Drug Users	Heterosexual Adults	High-Risk Youth	MSM	People Living with HIV/AIDS
Many Men, Many Voices (3MV)	—	×	—	—	—	×	—
Modelo de Intervencion Psicomedica (MIP)	—	×	×	—	—	—	—
Motivational Interviewing-based HIV Risk Reduction	—	×	×	×	—	—	—
Mpowerment	—	×	—	—	—	×	—
Nia	—	×	—	×	—	—	—
No Excuses/Sin Buscar Excusas	—	×	—	—	—	×	—
Options/Opciones Project	—	×	—	—	—	—	×
Partnership for Health	×	×	—	—	—	×	×
Personalized Cognitive Counseling (PCC)	—	×	—	—	—	×	—
Popular Opinion Leader (POL)	—	×	—	—	—	×	—
Positive Choice: Interactive Video Doctor	—	×	—	—	—	×	×
Preventing AIDS through Live Movement and Sound (PALMS)	—	×	—	—	×	—	—
Prime Time	—	×	—	—	×	—	—
Project FIO (The Future is Ours)	—	×	—	×	—	—	—
Project HEART	×	—	—	×	—	—	—
Project Image	—	×	—	—	×	—	—
Project START	—	×	—	×	—	—	—
RAPP	—	×	—	×	—	—	—
Real AIDS Prevention Project (RAPP)	—	×	—	×	—	—	—
REAL Men	—	×	—	—	×	—	—

Real Men Are Safe (REMAS)	—	×	×	—	—	—	—
RESPECT	—	×	×	×	—	—	—
SAFE	—	×	—	×	—	—	—
Safe in the City	—	×	—	×	×	—	—
Safe on the Outs	—	×	—	—	×	—	—
Safer Sex	—	×	—	—	×	—	—
Safer Sex Skills Building (SSSB)	—	×	×	×	—	—	—
SafeTalk	—	×	—	×	—	×	×
Safety Counts	—	×	×	—	—	—	—
Self-Help In Eliminating Life-Threatening Diseases (SHIELD)	—	×	×	—	—	—	—
Seropositive Urban Men's Initiative (SUMIT)	—	×	—	—	×	×	×
SEPA	—	×	—	×	—	—	—
SHIELD	—	×	×	—	—	—	—
Sistering, Informing, Healing, Living, and Empowering (SiHLE)	—	×	—	—	×	—	—
SISTA	—	×	—	—	×	—	—
Sisters Saving Sisters	—	×	—	—	×	—	—
Sister to Sister	—	×	—	×	—	—	—
SMART Couples	×	—	—	×	—	×	—
Sniffer	—	×	×	—	—	—	—
START	—	×	—	×	—	—	—
Street Smart	—	×	—	—	×	—	—
Strong African American Families-Teen (SAAF-T)	—	×	—	—	×	—	—
Study to Reduce Intravenous Exposures (STRIVE)	—	×	×	—	×	—	—
Teen Health	—	×	—	—	×	—	—

(continued on next page)

Table 1
(continued)

Intervention Name	Intervention Type		Risk Category				
	Medication Adherence	Behavioral Risk Reduction	Drug Users	Heterosexual Adults	High-Risk Youth	MSM	People Living with HIV/AIDS
Think Twice	—	×	—	—	—	×	—
Together Learning Choices (TLC)	—	×	—	—	×	×	×
Treatment Advocacy Program (TAP)	—	×	—	—	—	×	×
VOICES/VOCES	—	×	—	×	—	—	—
WILLOW	—	×	—	×	—	—	×
Women's Health Promotion (WHP)	—	×	—	×	—	—	—
Women's Co-Op	—	×	×	×	—	—	—
Young Men's Health Project	—	×	—	—	—	×	—

cost-effective, and have cost-saving outcomes by reducing future medical care expenses. CDPs have positively and significantly impacted sexual risk behaviors, thereby reducing risk for HIV and other STIs, especially among groups experiencing disproportionate HIV burden.[25] One campaign targeting sex workers solicited the support of brothel owners, sex workers, and their customers to increase condom access and use and to shift norms about condom use in the environment.[24,26]

Successful, effective, large-scale CDPs have been implemented by New York City's Department of Health and Mental Hygiene and the District of Columbia's Department of Health HIV/AIDS, Hepatitis, STD, and TB administration. The CDC recommends including the following elements for implementing an effective structural-level CDP[26]:

- Provide free condoms
- Have a wide distribution coverage area in traditional and nontraditional venues
- Promote condom use through social marketing campaigns; messages should raise awareness about the benefits of condoms and normalize condom use in communities
- Supplement CDP with intensive individual-level risk-reduction interventions and community-level interventions

Needle exchange

Harm-reduction programs distributing clean needles and syringes are another effective structural intervention to reduce HIV incidence among intravenous drug users. The World Health Organization recommendation is to provide 200 clean needles and syringes for each IDU per year. In addition to needle exchange,[27] other strategies to reducing HIV transmitted via needle-sharing include the following:

- Supplying equipment to prepare and consume drugs (ie, filters, mixing containers, sterile water)
- Teaching safer injection practices and strategies for avoiding and managing a drug overdose
- Teaching safe strategies for handling and disposing of drug injection equipment
- Providing referrals for HIV testing and treatment services
- Providing access to drug treatment and other health care services[28]

Amendments to the Connecticut state law requiring a physician prescription for clean needles and syringes positively impacted IDU and police officers who were susceptible to needle-stick injuries while working.[28] Research-based results of the policy change included the following[6]:

- Decrease in self-reported needle-sharing among IDU
- Fewer IDU purchasing syringes on the street
- Increase in IDU purchasing syringes from pharmacies
- Decrease in needle-stick injury rates among police officers

These harm-reduction strategies targeting HIV transmission via needle-sharing are cost effective and reduce HIV transmission without increasing intravenous drug use among individuals or in communities.[27]

SUMMARY

With no available cure for HIV, primary prevention to reduce the likelihood of HIV transmission and secondary prevention to reduce the severity of HIV by identifying cases early and quickly engaging people in the care continuum are key factors to reducing morbidity. Evidence-based and evidence-informed interventions are available to reduce disease incidence and disease burden. Although there are evidence-driven interventions available for people who are drug users, heterosexual adults, MSM, high-risk adolescents and young adults, and people living with HIV/AIDS, there are not currently any curricula addressing people with SMI. The next steps in HIV prevention must include disseminating and implementing evidence-based interventions to reduce HIV risk behavior, increase medication adherence, and link people with HIV/AIDS to the care continuum.

REFERENCES

1. Hall HI, An Q, Tang T, et al. Prevalence of diagnosed and undiagnosed HIV infection–United States, 2008-2012. MMWR Morb Mortal Wkly Rep 2015;64(24): 657–62. DCOM-20150904 (1545-861X (Electronic)).
2. CDC. HIV among African Americans. 2015. Available at: http://www.cdc.gov/hiv/group/racialethnic/africanamericans/index.html. Accessed June 15, 2015.
3. CDC. HIV Incidence. 2015.
4. CDC. Transmission. 2015. Available at: http://www.cdc.gov/hiv/basics/transmission.html. Accessed June 15, 2015.
5. CDC. Prevention. 2015. Available at: http://www.cdc.gov/hiv/basics/prevention.html. Accessed June 15, 2015.
6. Groseclose SL, Weinstein B, Jones TS, et al. Impact of increased legal access to needles and syringes on practices of injecting-drug users and police officers–Connecticut, 1992-1993. J Acquir Immune Defic Syndr Hum Retrovirol 1995; 10(1):82–9. DCOM-19950928 (1077-9450 (Print)).
7. Prince JD, Walkup J, Akincigil A, et al. Serious mental illness and risk of new HIV/AIDS diagnoses: an analysis of Medicaid beneficiaries in eight states. Psychiatr Serv 2013;63(10):1032–8. DCOM-20130530 (1557–9700 (Electronic)).
8. Brown LK, Tolou-Shams M, Lescano C, et al. Depressive symptoms as a predictor of sexual risk among African American adolescents and young adults. J Adolesc Health 2006;39(3):444.e1–8, 0821 DCOM-20061024 (1879–1972 (Electronic)).
9. Substance Abuse and Mental Health Services Administration (US). Treatment improvement protocol (TIP) series: chapter 4—primary and secondary HIV prevention. Center for Substance Abuse Treatment. Substance abuse treatment for persons with HIV/AIDS. Rockville (MD): Substance Abuse and Mental Health Services Administration (US); 2000.
10. Staton-Tindall M, Harp KL, Minieri A, et al. An exploratory study of mental health and HIV risk behavior among drug-using rural women in jail. Psychiatr Rehabil J 2015;38(1):45–54 (1559–3126 (Electronic)).
11. O'Cleirigh C, Traeger L, Mayer KH, et al. Anxiety specific pathways to HIV sexual transmission risk behavior among young gay and bisexual men. J Gay Lesbian Ment Health 2013;17(3):314–26 (1935-9705 (Print)).
12. Bradley H, Hall HI, Wolitski RJ, et al. Vital signs: HIV diagnosis, care, and treatment among persons living with HIV–United States, 2011. MMWR Morb Mortal Wkly Rep 2014;63(47):1113–7. DCOM-20150113.
13. Gross R, Bilker WB, Friedman HM, et al. Effect of adherence to newly initiated antiretroviral therapy on plasma viral load. AIDS 2001;15(16):2109–17. DCOM-20020118 (0269–9370 (Print)).
14. Reynolds NR, Testa MA, Marc LG, et al. Factors influencing medication adherence beliefs and self-efficacy in persons naive to antiretroviral therapy: a multi-center, cross-sectional study. AIDS Behav 2004;8:141–50. DCOM-20040818 (1090–7165 (Print)).

15. Chesney MA. Factors affecting adherence to antiretroviral therapy. Clin Infect Dis 2000;30(Suppl 2):S171–6.
16. Wu ES, Rothbard A, Holtgrave DR, et al. Determining the cost-savings threshold for HIV adherence intervention studies for persons with serious mental illness and HIV. Community Ment Health J 2014. [Epub ahead of print].
17. Walkup J, Blank MB, Gonzalez JS, et al. The impact of mental health and substance abuse factors on HIV prevention and treatment. J Acquir Immune Defic Syndr 2008;47(Suppl 1):S15–9. DCOM-20080429 (1525–4135 (Print)).
18. Wagner GJ, Kanouse DE, Koegel P, et al. Adherence to HIV antiretrovirals among persons with serious mental illness. AIDS Patient Care STDS 2003;17(4):179–86. DCOM-20030618 (1087–2914 (Print)).
19. CDC. Compendium of evidence-based interventions and best practices for HIV prevention. 2015. Available at: http://www.cdc.gov/hiv/prevention/research/compendium/lrc/index.html. Accessed September 18, 2015.
20. CDC. Behavioral interventions. Effective interventions: HIV prevention that works 2015. Available at: https://effectiveinterventions.cdc.gov/en/HighImpactPrevention/Interventions.aspx. Accessed September 18, 2015.
21. CDC. Medication adherence. Effective interventions: HIV prevention that works 2015. Available at: https://effectiveinterventions.cdc.gov/en/HighImpactPrevention/BiomedicalInterventions/MedicationAdherence.aspx. Accessed September 18, 2015.
22. CDC. Biomedical interventions. Effective interventions: HIV prevention that works 2015. Available at: https://effectiveinterventions.cdc.gov/en/HighImpactPrevention/BiomedicalInterventions.aspx. Accessed September 18, 2015.
23. Liau A, Crepaz N, Lyles CM, et al. Interventions to promote linkage to and utilization of HIV medical care among HIV-diagnosed persons: a qualitative systematic review, 1996-2011. AIDS Behav 2013;17:1941–62. DCOM-20130830 (1573-3254 (Electronic)).
24. University of California San Francisco (UCSF). What is the role of structural interventions in HIV prevention? University of California San Francisco (UCSF) Center for AIDS Prevention Studies; AIDS Research Institute; 2003.
25. CDC. Condom distribution programs. Effective interventions: HIV prevention that works 2015. Available at: https://effectiveinterventions.cdc.gov/en/HighImpactPrevention/StructuralInterventions/CondomDistribution.aspx. Accessed September 17, 2015.
26. CDC. Condom distribution as a structural level intervention. 2015. Available at: http://www.cdc.gov/hiv/prevention/programs/condoms/. Accessed September 17, 2015.
27. Avert. Needle and syringe programmes (NSPs) for HIV prevention. 2015. Available at: http://www.avert.org/needle-and-syringe-programmes-nsps-hiv-prevention.htm#footnote3_8yids81. Accessed September 10, 2015.
28. NICE. Needle and syringe programmes. 2015. Available at: http://www.nice.org.uk/guidance/ph52/resources/guidance-needle-and-syringe-programmes-pdf. Accessed September 10, 2015.

Substance Abuse Prevention

Sean R. LeNoue, MD[a,b,*], Paula D. Riggs, MD[c]

KEYWORDS

- Prevention • Substance abuse • Early intervention • School-based programs
- Substance use disorders • Risk factors

KEY POINTS

- Drug abuse is a common and prevalent problem among youth.
- Prevention interventions are classified as universal (population level), selective (targeting at-risk individuals), or indicated (targeting individuals showing early signs and symptoms of the illness).
- Additional research is needed to develop effective early and indicated interventions for youth at early stages of substance abuse.

INTRODUCTION

Research over the past 2 decades has clearly established substance use disorder (SUD) as a chronic, neurobiologically based medical illness with characteristics that are similar to other chronic medical conditions such as diabetes, asthma, obesity, and hypertension.[1] Advances in the treatment of many chronic medical conditions can be characterized generally by the development of more effective public education programs about risk and protective factors, systematic screening to identify at-risk individuals, and the development of more effective prevention and earlier interventions for individuals with early signs and symptoms of the illness. Progress in prevention and treatment of SUD has lagged behind progress in other areas of medicine. Substance abuse continues to account for nearly 6% of all deaths worldwide.[2] In the United States alone, the annual economic burden incurred through loss of work productivity,

Disclosure Statement/Conflicts of Interest: Dr S.R. LeNoue and Dr P.D. Riggs have no conflicts to disclose.
[a] University of Colorado School of Medicine, 13001 East 17th Place, Campus Box F546, Building 500, Room E2322, Aurora, CO 80045, USA; [b] Denver Health Medical Center, Department of Psychiatry, 777 Bannock Street, Mail Stop- 0490, Denver, CO 80204, USA; [c] Division of Substance Dependence, Department of Psychiatry, University of Colorado School of Medicine, Building 400, Mail Stop F478, Aurora, CO 80045, USA
* Corresponding author. University of Colorado School of Medicine, 13001 East 17th Place, Campus Box F546, Building 500, Room E2322, Aurora, CO 80045.
E-mail address: sean.lenoue@ucdenver.edu

Child Adolesc Psychiatric Clin N Am 25 (2016) 297–305
http://dx.doi.org/10.1016/j.chc.2015.11.007
1056-4993/16/$ – see front matter © 2016 Elsevier Inc. All rights reserved.

Abbreviations	
CBT	Cognitive–behavioral therapy
EFC	Educational feedback control
MET	Motivational enhancement therapy
SUD	Substance use disorder
TND	Project toward no drug abuse

health care expenses, and crime secondary to substance abuse is estimated to be more than $700 billion.[3]

Approximately 4 out of 5 drug users begin using during adolescence, and it is estimated that approximately 11% of adolescents meet diagnostic criteria for a SUD before age 18.[4] Alcohol continues to be the most widely used substance among adolescents with almost 25% of high school seniors reporting at least 1 episode of binge drinking ($\geq$5 drinks on 1 occasion) in the past 2 weeks and nearly 40% reporting illicit drug use in the past year. Although there have been gradual decreases in the prevalence of cigarette smoking and alcohol use since the mid-1990s, rates of marijuana use and nonmedical prescription drug abuse have been increasing since 2009.[5] In 2014, more than 20% of high school seniors reported using marijuana regularly (at least monthly) and nearly 6% reported using daily or near daily.[5] Increases in adolescent marijuana use are thought to be connected to a growing national support for the legalization of medical and recreational marijuana. The majority of adults and adolescents believe that regular marijuana use causes little harm.[5] This perception is in contrast to research showing that regular marijuana use during adolescence—a time of rapid brain development—is associated with persistent neurocognitive deficits and reductions in adult IQ that may not be fully reversible, even with abstinence.[6–9] Regular marijuana use during adolescence is also associated with lower overall academic achievement, higher rates of high school dropout, lower rates of college entrance and completion, as well as higher unemployment or underemployment in adulthood.[10]

The enormous public health impact of substance abuse, which typically begins during adolescence, highlights the importance of effective youth substance use prevention and treatment. Prevention science differentiates 3 types of prevention interventions: (1) universal or population-based strategies that affect everyone, (2) selective interventions for at-risk groups, and (3) indicated prevention for youth who have high-risk behaviors, including substance use or problematic use.[11,12] Most existing substance prevention programs include psychoeducational components and skills-based learning to reduce factors and increase protective factors.

Although a comprehensive review of drug/alcohol prevention interventions is beyond the scope of this article, representative drug/alcohol prevention interventions that have substantial empirical support are discussed.

SCHOOL-BASED PREVENTION STRATEGIES

The majority of existing prevention interventions are school-based programs because schools are an efficient way of reaching a large number of students across multiple grade levels.

Universal School-based Prevention

In the school setting, universal prevention typically includes substance awareness education and school-wide adoption of specific behavioral management programs that teach social and peer resistance skills and promote the development of positive peer affiliations.[13] Some offer specific curricula designed for implementation by teachers in classroom settings. Current research indicates the most effective prevention programs use a combination of teacher and nonteacher facilitators (eg, health workers and/or mental health counselors).[13] Overall, universal prevention interventions have a relatively small effect size on preventing or delaying the onset of substance use, but can result in significant reductions in government spending over the lifetime of an individual.[14–18]

A recent Cochrane review identified only 3 prevention interventions with sufficient empirical support to be deemed efficacious: (1) the Unplugged Program, (2) the Life Skills Program, and (3) the Good Behavior Game.[13] These universal school-based prevention interventions, discussed in more detail elsewhere in this paper, are intended for school-wide adoption and designed to reduce risk behaviors and promote positive prosocial behavior in all students.

The unplugged program
The Unplugged Program is a universal school-based substance abuse prevention program, developed for the European Drug Addiction Prevention Trial.[19,20] "Unplugged" uses a comprehensive social influence approach incorporating life skills elements designed to delay or prevent the onset of substance use/misuse among junior high school students, ages 12 to 14.[21] "Unplugged" has been evaluated using a large cluster randomized trial, involving 9 centers, 170 schools, and approximately 7000 students in 7 European countries. The program focuses on educating youth on substance use risk and protective factors as well as promoting essential life skills (eg, coping strategies, effective communication, self-control, assertiveness, and problem solving).[22] The curriculum is designed for seventh- and eighth-grade students and is taught over the course of 12 one-hour sessions. At 18 months after the intervention, students who participated in the "Unplugged" intervention reported 38% fewer episodes of drunkenness and 26% less marijuana use in the past month compared with those who participated in usual classroom activities. Short-term reductions in tobacco use did not persist at the 18-month follow-up. However, fewer youth who were nonsmokers at the time of the intervention had started smoking 18 months after treatment, compared with controls.

The life skills training program
The Life Skills Training Program was developed by Botvin and colleagues[23–26] to provide a framework of prevention for SUDs for children and adolescents. The Life Skills Training curriculum is delivered by teachers and composed of 3 primary elements that teach drug resistance skills, personal self-management skills, and enhance general social functioning over the course of 15 sessions in the first year (third through sixth grades), with 10 additional booster sessions in the second year (sixth through eighth grades), and 5 sessions in the third year (ninth through twelfth grades). Compared with controls, youth who participated in the Life Skills Training intervention showed a 50% greater reduction in binge drinking at the 1- and 2-year follow-up and reported less tobacco, alcohol, and cannabis use at the 6-year follow-up.[23]

The good behavior game
The Good Behavior Game is a universal school-based prevention program delivered in the classroom setting by first and second grade elementary school teachers.[27] The intervention uses a behavioral skills training and modeling approach to promote prosocial behaviors and adaptive functioning skills from an early age. As young adults, youth who participated in the Good Behavior Game intervention had significantly

lower rates of smoking and drug and alcohol use disorders, antisocial personality disorder, delinquency and incarceration for violent crimes, suicidal ideation, and use of behavioral health services compared with students who participated in standard classroom activities.[27]

These 3 universal school-based interventions have been broadly adopted and disseminated. Effective implementation requires substantial training, resources, and school staff time. Recent research has focused on the development of less costly online or computer-assisted school-based prevention interventions that can be delivered with consistent fidelity and that require less teacher/professional training. CLIMATE is one such intervention that has shown promise. This universal school-based intervention for eighth-grade (middle school) students uses a 12-session, Internet-based curriculum designed to prevent, delay onset, or reduce alcohol and cannabis use.[28] At 6- and 12-months after the intervention, youth who completed the CLIMATE curriculum demonstrated greater knowledge of alcohol and cannabis and reported fewer episodes of weekly drinking and intoxication compared with controls who received the usual health class curriculum. Replication and longer term follow-up studies are needed.

Selective and Indicated School-based Prevention

There has been far less research and development of selective and indicated prevention interventions compared with the substantial body of research on universal school-based prevention programs. One of the few selective interventions that has been tested in multiple controlled trials is the Project Toward No Drug Abuse (TND). The TND program was developed to address gaps in selective substance prevention interventions by targeting at risk youth in both traditional and nontraditional school settings.[23,29] Composed of twelve 40- to 50-minute lessons, the Project TND curriculum is delivered in the classroom setting over 4 to 6 weeks by teachers who are trained and certified in the intervention. The curriculum includes motivational activities, social skills training, decision-making skills, and adaptive coping strategies to reduce risk of using tobacco, alcohol, cannabis, and other illicit drugs. Analysis of data from 3 controlled trials involving students attending Project TND schools shows a modest reduction in hard drug and alcohol use, but minimal to no effect on tobacco and cannabis use compared with control schools.

There is clearly a need for more effective, evidence-based "selective" prevention interventions for "at-risk" youth. However, there is an even greater need for effective school-based interventions for the growing number of middle and high school students with problematic substance use and the estimated 10% to 15% who would meet diagnostic criteria for a SUD.[5,30] In addressing this gap, the distinction between "indicated" prevention and "treatment" is not very useful or practical from a clinical standpoint. Currently, "indicated" prevention is conceptualized as most appropriate for youth with substance-related risk behaviors, including those who may have initiated or started "experimenting" with drugs or alcohol, whereas those meeting diagnostic criteria for a SUD should be referred to "treatment." Practically speaking, this means referring such youth to community-based substance treatment program. Many such programs provide evidence-based substance treatment modalities with proven effectiveness (eg, motivational enhancement therapy [MET]/cognitive–behavioral therapy [CBT], or family-based interventions including Functional Family Therapy, Brief Strategic Family Therapy, Multidimensional Family Therapy, Multi-systemic Therapy, and Adolescent Community Reinforcement Approach). However, most existing community-based substance treatment programs predominantly serve youth referred by the juvenile justice system, the largest third-party payer for such treatment nationwide. Thus, very few substance treatment options exist for the growing number of high school students with SUDs who are not (yet) involved with juvenile justice. Some researchers have started to address this gap by developing and testing brief 1 to 3 session interventions that use motivational enhancement and cognitive behavioral approaches.

Winters and Leitten[31] studied the role of a brief school-based motivational intervention incorporating self-change strategies. Students were recruited from a public high school system and eligible for study participation if meeting *Diagnostic and Statistical Manual of Mental Disorders* IV diagnostic criteria for substance abuse but not a substance dependence diagnosis. Seventy-nine students (ages 14–17) were randomized to 1 of 3 groups: (i) adolescent-only brief intervention (2 sessions of Motivational Interviewing and self-change strategies plus diagnostic assessment), (ii) adolescent-only brief intervention (2 sessions of Motivational Interviewing and self-change strategies plus diagnostic assessment), as well as another session with the parent, or (iii) a diagnostic assessment only control group. Upon the assessment at the 6-month follow-up, both brief intervention groups reported fewer drug use behaviors (ethanol and illicit substances) and substance-related negative consequences (eg, health, family, legal, social, and motor vehicle) compared with the assessment-only control group. The incorporation of a parent segment seemed to further augment the effectiveness of the brief intervention.

Walker and colleagues[32] developed and evaluated the *Teen Marijuana Check-up*, a brief school-based motivational enhancement intervention for non–treatment-seeking high school students using cannabis. Enrolled high school students, grades 9 through12 and between the ages of 14 and 19 who smoked cannabis were recruited from 6 Seattle-area high schools. Students were eligible for study participation if they reported smoking marijuana at least 9 out of the past 30 days at baseline. After completing a baseline questionnaire, 310 adolescents were randomized to 1 of 3 treatment groups:

i. MET;
ii. Educational feedback control (EFC); or
iii. Delayed feedback control (assessment only).

Participants assigned to MET and EFC were offered the opportunity to participate in up to 4 additional (optional) CBT sessions after completing their assigned MET (2 sessions) or EFC (2 sessions) brief intervention. Participants in all 3 groups were evaluated at baseline, 3 months, and 12 months. The primary outcome measures were number of days of self-reported cannabis use and associated negative consequences of use. Participation in additional treatment, including optional CBT sessions offered to MET and EFC groups, was also assessed. At 3-month follow-up, MET participants reported less cannabis use compared with the EFC group, and both MET and EFC reported less cannabis use and fewer negative consequences than the delayed feedback control group. The 3-month difference between MET and EFC did not persist at the 12-month follow-up, but the difference between both intervention groups and delayed feedback control persisted at the 1-year follow-up. Although posttreatment participation in additional optional CBT sessions treatment was minimal (offered to MET and EFC completers), there was a small but significant positive relationship between number of CBT sessions attended and decreased cannabis use.

Regardless of whether these brief school-based interventions are conceptualized as "indicated" prevention or early treatment these studies support, the feasibility, acceptability, and need for school-based interventions for high school students with cannabis and other SUDs. Taken together, results also suggest that 1 to 3 session interventions may be too brief to produce clinically meaningful and sustained reductions in substance use. Results of the study conducted by Walker and colleagues[32] are consistent with a larger and more substantial body of adolescent treatment research that suggests the combination of MET/CBT delivered over 6 to 12 sessions may be a more optimal dose of treatment for youth who have progressed to substance abuse or SUDs and is the modality most consistently associated with sustained or emerging treatment effects.[33]

NON–SCHOOL-BASED PREVENTION STRATEGIES
Universal Non–School-based Prevention

A 2006 Cochrane review of non–school-based drug prevention interventions concluded that there is currently a lack of evidence of the effectiveness of non–school-based interventions owing to methodological weaknesses including high rates of loss-to-follow up. The review found little empirical support for complex multicomponent community-based universal prevention interventions or psychoeducation, but did highlight 3 family interventions (eg, Preparing for the Drug Free Years and Iowa Strengthening Families Program are both universal preventive programs, whereas Focus on Families has elements of selective prevention for children and indicated prevention for adults) as showing some benefit for preventing self-reported cannabis use.[34,35]

Selective and Indicated Non–School-based Prevention

Although the aforementioned Cochrane review did not identify any non–school-based prevention interventions in any category (eg, universal, selective, indicated), it is important to highlight that several family-based interventions have been shown to be effective treatment for children and adolescents with conduct disorder and other serious behavior problems including antisocial behavior. These include Parent Management Training, Functional Family Therapy, Multidimensional Family Therapy, Brief Strategic Family Therapy, and Multisystemic Therapy. A subset of these (eg, Functional Family Therapy, Multidimensional Family Therapy, Brief Strategic Family Therapy, Multi-systemic Therapy) have also been shown to be effective treatments for adolescents with SUDs. Although a review of these family-based interventions is beyond the scope of this article, these and other interventions that reduce conduct and mental health problems (eg, attention deficit hyperactivity disorder, depression) that increase risk of adolescent substance abuse, can be conceptualized as "selective" or "indicated" drug/alcohol prevention interventions and are most often found in community-based mental health, substance treatment, or juvenile justice treatment settings.

In the context of national health care reforms, there has been greater interest regarding the potential benefits of universal drug/alcohol screening and prevention (behavioral counseling) in primary care medical settings. However, after rigorous review of current research, the 2015 US Prevention Services Task Force concluded that presently there is insufficient evidence to assess the benefits or potential harms of behavioral interventions to prevent or reduce adolescent alcohol, illicit drug, or prescription drug abuse in primary care medical settings.[36]

SUMMARY/DISCUSSION

Overall, prevention research has made significant progress in the development and implementation of effective universal, school-based drug/alcohol prevention programs including the Good Behavior Game, Unplugged, and Life Skills Training

Program. There would be significant benefit from policy and funding decisions to promote broader dissemination of these interventions. By contrast, progress has been slow, and there have been few research advances in developing effective "selective" and "indicated" prevention interventions. These gaps are further amplified against the backdrop of growing national concerns about problems related to adolescent drug and alcohol use and the inadequacy of the national treatment system to address these problems, given that only approximately 10% to 15% of adolescents who could benefit from substance treatment currently receive it.[5,36,37] Treatment options are extremely limited for the growing number of high school students with problematic substance use or who meet criteria for a SUD but who are not (yet) involved with the juvenile justice system. Additional research is needed to identify the most appropriate and effective interventions for such youth. Perhaps a good place to start would be well-designed studies of existing evidence-based substance treatment interventions (eg, MET/CBT) adapted as school-based interventions.

REFERENCES

1. McLellan AT, Lewis DC, O'Brien CP, et al. Drug dependence, a chronic medical illness: implications for treatment, insurance, and outcomes evaluations. JAMA 2000;284(13):1689–95.
2. World Health Organization (WHO). "Global status report on alcohol and health." Management of substance abuse - alcohol. Geneva (Switzerland): World Health Organization; 2012. Available at: www.who.int/substance_abuse/publications/global_alcohol_report/en/. Accessed August 2, 2015.
3. National Institute on Drug Abuse (NIDA). Substance abuse - trends and statistics. 2015. Available at: www.drugabuse.gov/related-topics/trends-statistics#costs. Accessed August 2, 2015.
4. Merikangas KR, He JP, Burstein M, et al. Lifetime prevalence of mental disorders in U.S. adolescents: results from the National Comorbidity Survey Replication–Adolescent Supplement (NCS-A). J Am Acad Child Adolesc Psychiatry 2010; 49(10):980–9.
5. Johnston LD, O'Malley PM, Miech RA, et al. Monitoring the future national survey results on drug use: 1975-2014: overview, key findings on adolescent drug use. Ann Arbor (MI): Institute for Social Research, The University of Michigan; 2015.
6. Brook JS, Stimmel MA, Zhang C, et al. The association between earlier marijuana use and subsequent academic achievement and health problems: a longitudinal study. Am J Addict 2008;17(2):155–60.
7. Pope HG, Gruber AJ, Hudson JI, et al. Cognitive measures in long-term cannabis users. J Clin Pharmacol 2002;42:41S–7S.
8. Meier MH, Caspi A, Ambler A, et al. Persistent cannabis users show neuropsychological decline from childhood to midlife. Proc Natl Acad Sci U S A 2012; 109:E2657–64.
9. Schneider M. Puberty as a highly vulnerable developmental period for the consequences of cannabis exposure. Addict Biol 2008;13:253–63.
10. Fergusson DM, Horwood J, Ridder EM. Conduct and attentional problems in childhood and adolescence and later substance use, abuse and dependence: results of a 25-year longitudinal study. Drug Alcohol Depend 2007;88(Suppl 1): S14–26.
11. Institute of Medicine. Reducing risks for mental disorders: frontiers for preventive intervention research. Washington, DC: National Academy Press; 1994.

12. National Research Council and Institute of Medicine. Preventing mental, emotional, and behavioral disorders among young people: progress and possibilities. Committee on the prevention of mental disorders and substance abuse among children, youth, and young adults: research advances and promising interventions. In: O'Connell ME, Boat T, Warner KE, editors. Board on children, youth, and families, division of behavioral and social sciences and education. Washington, DC: The National Academies Press; 2009. p. 6–10.

13. Foxcroft DR, Tsertsvadze A. Universal school-based prevention programs for alcohol misuse in young people. Evid Based Child Health 2012;7(2):450–575.

14. Caulkins JP, Pacula RL, Paddock S, et al. What we can - and cannot - expect from school-based drug prevention. Drug Alcohol Rev 2004;23:79–87.

15. DeWitt DJ, Adlaf EM, Offord DR, et al. Age at first alcohol use: a risk factor for the development of alcohol disorders. Am J Psychiatry 2000;157:745–50.

16. Pitkanen T, Lyyra AL, Pulkinnen L. Age of onset of drinking and the use of alcohol in adulthood: a follow-up study from age 8-42 for females and males. Addiction 2005;100:652–61.

17. Grant BF, Dawson DA. Age at onset of alcohol use and its association with DSM-IV alcohol abuse and dependence: results from the national longitudinal alcohol epidemiologic survey. J Subst Abuse 1997;9(1):103–10.

18. Grant BF, Dawson DA. Age of onset of drug use and its association with DSM-IV drug abuse and dependence: results from the national longitudinal alcohol epidemiologic survey. J Subst Abuse 1998;10(2):163–73.

19. Faggiano F, Galanti MR, Bohrn K, et al. The effectiveness of a school-based substance abuse prevention program: EU-dap cluster randomised controlled trial. Prev Med 2008;47:537–43.

20. Faggiano F, Vigna-Taglianti F, Burkhart G, et al. The effectiveness of a school-based substance abuse prevention program: 18-month follow-up of the EU-dap cluster randomized controlled trial. Drug Alcohol Depend 2010;108:56–64.

21. Sussman S, Earleywine M, Wills T, et al. The motivation, skills, and decision-making model of 'drug abuse' prevention. Subst Use Misuse 2004;39:1971–2016.

22. Caywood K, Riggs P, Novins D. Adolescent substance use disorder - prevention and treatment. Colorado Journal of Psychiatry and Psychology 2015;1:42–9.

23. Griffin KW, Botvin GJ. Evidence-based interventions for preventing substance use disorders in adolescents. Child Adolesc Psychiatr Clin N Am 2010;19(3):505–26.

24. Botvin G, Baker E, Renick N, et al. A cognitive-behavioral approach to substance abuse prevention. Addict Behav 1984;9:137–47.

25. Botvin G, Baker E, Dusenbury L, et al. Long-term follow-up results of a randomized drug abuse prevention trial in a white middle-class population. JAMA 1995; 273(14):1106–12.

26. Botvin G, Griffin K, Diaz T, et al. Preventing binge drinking during early adolescence: one- and two-year follow-up of a school-based preventive intervention. Psychol Addict Behav 2001;15(4):360–5.

27. Kellam SG, Mackenzie AC, Brown CH, et al. The good behavior game and the future of prevention and treatment. Addict Sci Clin Pract 2011;6(1):73–84.

28. Newton N, Teesson M, Vogl L, et al. Internet-based prevention for alcohol and cannabis use: final results of the climate schools course. Addiction 2009;105: 749–59.

29. Dent C, Sussman S, Stacy A. Project towards no drug abuse: generalizability to a general high school sample. Prev Med 2001;32:514–20.

30. Substance Abuse and Mental Health Services Administration. Results from the 2013 National Survey on Drug Use and Health: summary of national findings.

NSDUH Series H-48, HHS Publication No. (SMA) 14–4863. Rockville (MD): Substance Abuse and Mental Health Services Administration; 2014.

31. Winters KC, Leitten W. Brief intervention for drug abusing adolescents in a school setting. Psychol Addict Behav 2007;21(2):249–54.

32. Walker DD, Stephens R, Roffman R. Randomized controlled trial of motivational enhancement therapy with non-treatment-seeking adolescent cannabis users: a further test of the teen marijuana check-up. Psychol Addict Behav 2011;25(3): 474–84.

33. Tripodi SJ, Bender K, Litschge C, et al. Interventions for reducing adolescent alcohol abuse - a meta-analytic review. Arch Pediatr Adolesc Med 2010;164(1): 85–91.

34. Gates S, McCambridge J, Smith LA, et al. Interventions for prevention of drug use by young people delivered in non-school settings. Cochrane Database Syst Rev 2006;(1):CD005030.

35. Curry SJ, McNellis RJ. Behavioral counseling in primary care perspectives in enhancing the evidence base. Am J Prev Med 2015;49(3S2):S125–8.

36. McLellan AT, Meyers K. Contemporary addiction treatment: a review of systems problems for adults and adolescents. Biol Psychiatry 2004;56:764–70.

37. Substance Abuse Mental Health Services Administration (SAMHSA). Results from the 2010 national survey on drug use and health: summary of national findings. Rockville (MD): Substance Abuse and Mental Health Services Administration; 2011.

A Population Health Approach to System Transformation for Children's Healthy Development

 CrossMark

Paul H. Dworkin, MD[a],*, Aradhana Bela Sood, MD, MSHA[b,c]

KEYWORDS

- Child health services • Child development • Health promotion • Population health
- System transformation • Public policy • Social determinants • Child advocacy

KEY POINTS

- Achieving system transformation to promote children's healthy development requires public policy that contributes to and sustains long-term impact on population health.
- We must focus on promoting the healthy development of all children, as opposed to exclusively focusing on children with delays, disorders, and diseases.
- An integrated system of care is characterized by strong communication and collaboration across and among diverse sectors.
- System transformation must make optimal use of existing community resources.
- A strong evidence base and effective use of data must inform planning and advocacy.

According to the American Academy of Pediatrics, child health providers are "committed to the attainment of optimal physical, mental, and social health and well-being for all infants, children, adolescents, and young adults."[1] Despite this emphasis on promoting children's healthy development, much of the efforts of child health care providers are focused on maintaining wellness and treating illness. But what if we expanded child health services to not "merely" treat, or even prevent, diseases and disorders of individual children, but also to encompass the promotion of all children's optimal development? Advances in our knowledge of early brain development and early child development demand that we no longer view this question as rhetorical.

We declare no commercial or financial conflicts of interest or funding sources for this work.
[a] Department of Pediatrics, Office for Community Child Health, *Help Me Grow* National Center, Connecticut Children's Medical Center, University of Connecticut School of Medicine, 282 Washington Street, Hartford, CT 06106, USA; [b] Department of Psychiatry, Virginia Commonwealth University, 515 N 10th Street, Richmond, VA 23298, USA; [c] Department of Pediatrics, Virginia Commonwealth University, 515 N 10th Street, Richmond, VA 23298, USA
* Corresponding author.
E-mail address: pdworki@connecticutchildrens.org

Child Adolesc Psychiatric Clin N Am 25 (2016) 307–317
http://dx.doi.org/10.1016/j.chc.2015.12.004
1056-4993/16/$ – see front matter © 2016 Elsevier Inc. All rights reserved.

childpsych.theclinics.com

More recently, our enhanced understanding of the impact of toxic stress and the biology of adversity, including the "biological embedding of environmental events" and the extent to which chronic stress affects the body's physiologic systems (ie, cardiovascular, neuroendocrine, and immune), requires us to address the myriad of psychosocial factors, so-called social determinants of health, that increase vulnerability to a wide range of disorders.[2] In this article, we explore implications from the science of early brain/early child development and childhood adversity and toxic stress for system building to promote children's healthy development. We provide examples of public policy that enable system transformation in support of population health. We share the story of *Help Me Grow*, designed to support children's flourishing across a range of developmental trajectories, to illustrate the characteristics of successful system transformation. *Help Me Grow* is an evidence-based intervention that focuses on the linking of children and their families to community-based programs and services to strengthen protective factors that promote children's optimal healthy development. Finally, we explore implications from the *Help Me Grow* experience for population health system transformation and public policy.

THE SCIENTIFIC RATIONALE FOR SYSTEM TRANSFORMATION

The explosion in our knowledge of early brain development and early child development, so rapidly accelerated as a consequence of advancing technologies such as brain imaging (eg, functional MRI) and brain functioning (eg, brain electrical activity mapping [BEAM]), inspired the widespread public and professional dissemination of findings in the 1990s, the so-called "decade of the brain." These advances in our knowledge have yielded important implications for our interventions to promote children's healthy development. The complexities and opportunities of early child development demand that we shift our focus from the efficacy of such specific services and programs as child health services and early intervention to the design and implementation of comprehensive population health systems that engage multiple sectors in promoting all children's developmental flourishing.

Examples of concepts in early brain development informing interventions to promote children's healthy development include proportional brain growth, neural plasticity, critical periods, sequential development, and the role of experience. Although detailed explanations are beyond the scope of this article, the understanding that brain growth disproportionately occurs during the prenatal period and earliest years of life; that neural plasticity, although an enduring attribute of the nervous system across the life span, offers greatest opportunities during the early years; that certain stimuli are necessary during critical periods of early life to ensure normal brain development (eg, consider the permanent impairment of vision if a newborn is unable to process visual stimuli due to a congenital cataract); that development is sequential and stimuli must also be sequential (eg, few infants will benefit from an algebra lesson and few adolescents need to be held each day); and the role of early experience in shaping brain structure and function.[3] The latter concept, in particular, lends itself to vivid illustration. At birth, there are 50 trillion synapses among the neurons of the brain. With appropriate exposure to a variety of development-enhancing stimuli, the number of synapses increases 20-fold to 1000 trillion by 1 year of age.[4] Enriching experiences during the duration of childhood enable the brain to eliminate those synapses unhelpful or unnecessary through the process of pruning in the period broadly described as adolescence, thereby achieving efficiency and capacity, such that by early adulthood the number of synapses has been halved to some 500 trillion. At each stage in the process, the remolded brain facilitates the embrace of new experiences, and so goes the process.

These critical concepts in early brain development have obvious yet profound implications for our interventions:

- For optimal effectiveness, services must begin as early as possible during infancy;
- Stimulation during the first 3 years of life is particularly critical to ensure optimal development, given the realities of critical periods and neural plasticity. Although the latter does not constitute a "use it or lose it" imperative, the unparalleled ability during the early years of life to influence neural changes in the brain demand our attention; and
- Given the implications of critical periods and sequential development, services must be both comprehensive and appropriately aligned with children's developmental stages and needs.
- The focus of this article is on setting the trajectory of development on an optimum course in early childhood by programs supporting healthy brain development. However, opportunities for later prevention efforts during adolescence should not be underestimated. This is a period of major architectural reshaping of the brain for neurobehavioral efficiency, when the emergence of major mental illnesses coexist with opportunities for enhancing resilience.

A number of critical concepts in early child development similarly have profoundly important implications for system transformation. Although a comprehensive iteration of such concepts is beyond the scope of this review, several deserve mention. Neal Halfon, Director of the University of California Los Angeles Center for Healthier Children, Families, and Communities, has described the utility of viewing children as progressing along developmental or school readiness trajectories.[5] Most of our clinical and policy attention is directed at children progressing along a disordered/delayed trajectory. Fortunately, most children progress along a healthy trajectory, albeit manifesting a wide range of normal skills and abilities. Halfon and Hochstein[5] also identify a group of children progressing along an at-risk trajectory, for whom positive circumstances and experiences may ultimately enable ascent to a healthy trajectory or, more commonly, adverse experiences may result in deterioration to a delayed/disordered trajectory. At any given age, a variety of factors, both favorable and unfavorable, influence children's development. Examples of facilitative factors include parent education, parent emotional health, a protective home environment, access to a medical home, high-quality early care and education programs, and neighborhood safety and support. In contrast, such adverse social determinants as poverty, lack of access to health services, and exposure to domestic violence impair children's developmental well-being.[5] Chamberlin[6] described the implications of developmental trajectories for interventions that promote children's developmental flourishing in noting that, "the most effective long-term strategy appears to be the development of a comprehensive, community-wide approach focused on preventing low- and medium-risk families from becoming high-risk, as well as providing intensive services to those who already have reached a high-risk status." Halfon and Hochstein[5] also point out that interventions for such low-risk and medium-risk children are typically more accessible and efficacious than those focused on children with delays and disorders.

Our understanding of factors both promoting and hindering children's optimal healthy development is informed by critical research on social determinants of health; for example, those conditions into which we are born, grow, live, and age. The World Health Organization Commission on Social Determinants of Health describes both structural determinants (eg, socioeconomic, political, and governance structures) and an individual's place relating to race, ethnicity, gender, and class, as well as intermediary health determinants (ie, a broad range of working and living conditions, behavior and biology, and other psychosocial factors affecting the individual within a community).[7] McGinnis and colleagues[8] attribute 90% of health outcomes to social/environmental, genetic, and behavioral factors. Social determinants of health importantly contribute to health disparities and inequities, emphasizing the imperative that comprehensive system building engage sectors beyond health care. Research on the correlation between social determinants and mental health outcomes confirms that the implications for policy and system building are likely of similar importance for behavioral health.[9]

These critical concepts have important implications for system transformation:

- Treatment programs and services must be comprehensive, multidisciplinary, and address the multiple factors that facilitate and hinder children's optimal development;
- Services should address the needs of all children; for example, the entire population, recognizing that those in greatest need will likely derive the greatest benefit. We must expand our target population to all children, especially to vulnerable, at-risk children and their families, while recognizing the limitations of an exclusive focus on children with complex disorders and delays; and
- System building must engage all sectors so important to promoting family resiliency, enhancing protective factors, and promoting children's healthy development. Examples include but are not necessarily limited to the sectors of child health services, early care and education, family support, child welfare, food and nutrition, neighborhood health and safety, healthy homes, transportation, workforce development and employment, economic development, arts and culture, and faith-based initiatives.

PUBLIC POLICY, POPULATION HEALTH, AND SYSTEM TRANSFORMATION

Achieving system transformation to promote children's healthy development requires public policy that contributes to and sustains long-term impact on population health.[10] Select examples of such policy include promoting the healthy development of all children, as opposed to exclusively focusing on children with delays, disorders, and diseases; creating an integrated system of care with strong communication and collaboration across and among diverse sectors; making optimal use of existing community resources; and building a strong evidence base and effectively using data to inform planning and advocacy.

Promote the Healthy Development of all Children

Federal and state programs (eg, Part C and Part B of the Individuals with Disabilities Education Act [IDEA], Title V funding for Children and Youth with Special Health Care Needs [CYSHCN]) require children to fulfill specific eligibility criteria to receive services and supports. Although addressing the needs of children with delays and disorders, such eligibility criteria typically fail to include vulnerable children progressing along an at-risk trajectory, despite the benefits of their linkage to community-based interventions. Expanding the focus of early detection and intervention efforts to include vulnerable children at risk for adverse developmental and behavioral outcomes will maximize value and societal impact. Corollaries to this principle include supporting community-based efforts that promote the health and safety of children in a variety of settings and expanding those activities that identify and address children's needs as early as possible.

Create Integrated Systems of Care with Strong Linkages

Comprehensive system building must engage the key sectors so important to the well-being of families and their children and ensure cross-sector collaboration and communication. For example, policies should encourage partnerships across such sectors as child health services, early care and education, and family support services to ensure effective developmental promotion, early detection, and the linkage of children and their families to community-based programs and services. Early detection is facilitated by policies that embed the process of developmental surveillance and screening into the full spectrum of services that young children use across these sectors. Furthermore, ensuring that early detection leads to assessment and intervention will contribute to children's optimal healthy development. Connecting community-based programs and services to each other can decrease duplication and streamline services for families.

Make Optimal Use of Existing Resources

Policy makers are understandably mindful of budget challenges at the levels of federal and local jurisdictions and are often reluctant to support initiatives that impose additional financial burdens. A variety of strategies ensures the efficient use of existing resources, while not necessarily demanding an increase in expenditures. Examples include elevating the role of care coordination in accessing services within and across sectors, strengthening the effectiveness of child health services to make an optimal contribution to children's healthy development, identifying ways to achieve cost efficiencies through the blending of administrative and financial resources of departments and agencies, documenting short-term and longer-term cost savings from various interventions, and using linkage of children and their families to community-based programs and services to demonstrate real-time cost-effectiveness.[11]

Build a Strong Evidence Base and Use Data More Effectively

Policies enabling the use of data to document gaps and capacity issues serve to inform advocacy and to emphasize the need to strengthen child health and community services. Data collection and analysis are critical to demonstrating the efficacy of innovations and justifying their funding. Given the challenges of demonstrating the efficacy of interventions through advances in children's developmental status, polices should endorse the application of mediating factors, such as family resiliency, that are important determinants of developmental outcomes. Policies should minimize or eliminate barriers to developing system performance measures and data sets, which may include sharing or integrating data across agencies and sectors to establish a comprehensive resource and referral database, coordinate care, and monitor outcomes.

THE *HELP ME GROW* STORY

Our experience with a community-based approach to promoting the flourishing of vulnerable children at risk for developmental and behavioral problems demonstrates the application of key public policy concepts and offers implications for system transformation. In the mid-1990s, with support and encouragement from a local foundation, the Hartford Foundation for Public Giving's (HFPG) Brighter Futures initiative, child health providers considered how to better meet the needs of Hartford, Connecticut's children and families to promote children's flourishing and optimal developmental outcomes. Planning partners included the City Health Department and its Child Development Program, parent groups, child health advocates, community-based organizations, elected officials, and the state's early intervention program, Birth to Three. Discussions yielded shared assumptions that led to the design of *Help Me Grow*:

- Children with developmental and behavioral problems were eluding early detection;
- Even in resource-challenged Hartford, many initiatives existed to provide services to young children and their families;
- A gap existed between child health services and child development and early childhood education programs; and
- Hartford's children and their families would benefit from a coordinated, region-wide system of early detection and care coordination.

The design of *Help Me Grow* includes 4 core components:

- Training child health providers, parents, and other key informants in effective developmental surveillance and screening to promote early detection[12];
- Creating a computerized resource inventory of regional programs and services promoting developmental flourishing and addressing the developmental and behavioral needs of children and their families;
- Establishing a triage, referral, and care coordination system, Child Development Infoline, to facilitate access to services and support; and
- Systematically gathering data on the developmental status and needs of children to identify gaps in services and advocate for measures to close such gaps.[13]

HFPG supported a pilot study of *Help Me Grow* in Hartford from 1997 to 2002. The documented effectiveness of *Help Me Grow* in enhancing the early detection of urban Hartford's vulnerable children and the linkage of these children and their families to developmentally enhancing programs and services informed and supported the advocacy that led to its incorporation within the state budget and its dissemination as a statewide program of the Connecticut Children's Trust Fund in 2002.[14] The advocacy resulting in successful statewide dissemination of *Help Me Grow* in Connecticut demanded securing the attention of the early childhood development policy subsystem, including executive and legislative branches of government, state agencies, interest groups, scientists and academicians, the media, and the general public. Connecticut's public programs addressing developmental delays and disorders, including Birth to Three, Preschool Special Education, and the Children and Youth with Special Healthcare Needs Program (Title V of the Social Security Act), each have restrictive eligibility criteria that require evidence of significant delays and disorders and do not allow a focus on vulnerable children at risk of developmental and behavioral problems. For many years, efforts to expand eligibility criteria failed and the state, popularly known as the "land of steady habits," displayed no propensity to altering its priorities or stance on this issue. Thus, advocacy in support of expansion of eligibility for state programs and services was figuratively "dead on the legislative doorstep." In contrast, changing the content of communication and portraying *Help Me Grow* as a strategy to enhance the access of vulnerable children and their families to community-based programs and services (eg, family resource centers, parenting programs, child care), typically at no cost to the state, received enthusiastic support.

The securing of executive branch support illustrates the benefit of such "strategic framing." In early 2000, coincident with advocacy efforts in support of *Help Me Grow* dissemination, then Governor John Rowland actively supported a statewide initiative, Connecticut Community KidCare, designed to reform the manner in which children's behavioral health services are coordinated, financed, and delivered.[15]

A key priority of the initiative was to enable more children with complex behavioral health needs to receive services in their community. Coincidentally, analysis of the Hartford-based *Help Me Grow* pilot program documented the high prevalence of referrals of children whose parents have concerns for their behavior.[14] These data enabled the framing of *Help Me Grow* as a behavioral health program that served at-risk children to prevent the escalation of behavioral concerns to mental health disorders, thereby essentially serving as the prevention component of Connecticut Community KidCare. The governor enthusiastically received this proposal and included support for statewide dissemination of *Help Me Grow* in his 2002 budget proposal, with subsequent endorsement by the legislature.

Annual evaluation documents that *Help Me Grow* fulfills state requirements for results-based accountability, thereby enabling sustained budget support.[16] For example, since 2002, 85% of children and families referred to Connecticut's *Help Me Grow* have been successfully connected with community-based programs and services.[17] Although successful linkage of children and their families to developmental programs and services is a key process measure, the impact of *Help Me Grow* on children's healthy development is an important outcome measure. However, the outcome of interest, for example, enhanced child development, raises formidable measurement issues. The myriad of influences on children's developmental outcomes and the multiple reasons for so-called "downstream effects" challenge efforts to demonstrate the relationship between program penetration and the developmental status of children within the target population.[18] The difficulties inherent in attempting to ascribe developmental outcomes to any single, specific intervention, such as support from *Help Me Grow*, are circumvented by, instead, focusing on subobjectives.[3] Research has examined the extent to which the programs and services to which *Help Me Grow* links children and their families enhance 5 protective factors that are known to correlate with positive developmental outcomes, the foundation of the Strengthening Families Approach of the Center for the Study of Social Policy.[19] Through referral and linkage to community-based programs and services, *Help Me Grow* enhances parental resilience, social connections, concrete support in times of need, knowledge of parenting and child development, and children's social and emotional competence.[20] Cost-benefit analyses of *Help Me Grow*, as evidence of the efficiency of the program, are also important in supporting requests for foundation and public funding. For example, *Help Me Grow* decreases reliance on referrals to medical specialists and facilitates connections to community-based, lower-cost programs and services.[11]

In 2007, the founders of *Help Me Grow* provided informal guidance to Orange County, California, to enable replication of the system in that county. From 2008 to 2010, a grant from The Commonwealth Fund to the founders supported the provision of technical assistance to 5 states desiring to replicate *Help Me Grow*. In 2010, support from the W.K. Kellogg Foundation established the *Help Me Grow* National Center at Connecticut Children's Medical Center in Hartford, and provided the resources to continue replication efforts within the original 5 states and engage an additional 10 states over 3 years as affiliates, with the goal of enabling 15 states (plus Connecticut) to develop *Help Me Grow* systems. At present, more than 25 states and territories are affiliates of the National Center.[21]

The success of *Help Me Grow* replication is predicated on fidelity to the model, including the previously described 4 core components, as well as 3 structural requirements, including an organizing entity, a strategy for expanding statewide over time, and the capacity and commitment to implement a process for continuous quality improvement (**Fig. 1**). Other key attributes of *Help Me Grow* integral to its success include the following:

- A focus on the developmental flourishing of all children, especially those vulnerable and at risk for adverse developmental and behavioral outcomes;
- The promotion of developmental surveillance and screening as the optimal process for early detection;
- The provision of a central portal of entry to developmental and behavioral programs and services;
- The promotion of cross-sector collaboration among child health services, early care and education, and family support services;
- The commitment to blend administrative and financial resources across state agencies and programs (including IDEA, Part C and B services);
- The facilitation of data sharing; and
- The embedding of *Help Me Grow* within related initiatives to enhance both replication and sustainability. For example, states have now integrated *Help Me Grow* within a variety of federal initiatives, including Maternal, Infant, and Early Childhood Home Visiting Programs (Health Resources and Services Administration), Race to the Top-Early Learning Challenge (US Department of Education), Learn the Signs. Act Early (Centers for Disease Control and Prevention), and Project LAUNCH (Substance Abuse and Mental Health Services Administration).

IMPLICATIONS FOR EFFECTIVE SYSTEM TRANSFORMATION

Our experience emphasizes the importance of considering interventions in the context of a system transformation strategy, as opposed to a focus on individual programs or services. An example is strengthening the capacity of child health providers to perform early detection through the process of developmental surveillance and screening. Although changes in provider practice may increase the number of children identified to be at risk for poor developmental outcomes, developmental trajectories will not be improved unless such detection leads to referral and, ultimately, linkage to community-based programs and services. Such system-wide characteristics as care coordination capacity and the availability of appropriate programs are as essential as effective early detection practices.

Despite the importance of child health services as a platform for developmental promotion, early detection, and referral to services, the myriad of available interventions

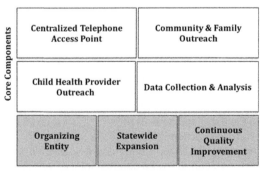

Fig. 1. Core components and structural requirements of *Help Me Grow*.

to promote children's healthy development mainly reside within such human services sectors as early care and education and family support. Furthermore, crucial neighborhood-level and household-level social determinants of children's healthy development involve many additional sectors critical to system building.[22] Examples include, but are not limited to, healthy homes, safe neighborhoods, child welfare, workforce development, food and nutrition, transportation, economic development, arts and culture, and faith-based initiatives. Cross-sector collaboration is essential to address families' needs in a comprehensive and integrated fashion. The concept of medical home should be reframed as a health neighborhood to acknowledge the importance of community-based programs and services beyond the purview of child health providers.[23]

Health care reform's relentless pursuit of return on investment and so-called "scorable savings" has encouraged a focus on the subset of children with complex medical conditions who most heavily consume medical services and account for most Medicaid expenditures.[24] However, an exclusive focus on such children fails to acknowledge the well-documented benefits of targeting the needs of all children, that is, a population health approach, especially those most vulnerable children at risk for developmental and behavioral problems. Interventions for all children, such as parenting classes, home visiting, and high-quality child care, are often widely available, accessible, efficacious, and cost-effective.

Referrals should not be equated with successful linkage to programs and services, as research demonstrates that vulnerable children and their families frequently fail to receive recommended interventions.[25] *Help Me Grow* demonstrates how access to interventions is facilitated by a central portal of entry requiring a single call to a care coordinator staffing an information and referral service. Blending administrative and financial resources across services and sectors strengthens care coordination capacity, efficiency, and effectiveness, facilitating families' access to interventions by overcoming barriers and acknowledging families' frequent needs for guidance and support. A centralized process of referral also enables data collection, both to demonstrate the efficacy of the linkage process and to gather information on important gaps and capacity issues to inform advocacy and planning.

We conclude that our still-evolving knowledge of early brain/child development, social determinants of health, and the biology of adversity demands that we redefine the content and process of interventions to promote children's healthy development. Successful interventions, such as *Help Me Grow*, are best viewed in the context of comprehensive systems supporting all children's developmental flourishing. For examples of interventions applying similar, key social policy principles see: Hudziak JJ, Ivanova M. The Vermont family-based approach: family-based health promotion, illness prevention, and intervention, in this issue. VFBA expands the focus of child psychiatry assessment and treatment from illness to wellness and from the individual child to the entire family environment. Halfon and Hochstein's[5] Life Course Health Development model has been used to inform new approaches to health promotion, disease prevention, and developmental optimization by redesigning the delivery and financing of health care.

We must expand our focus beyond that of children with complex medical conditions, delays, and disorders to a population health approach that ensures that all children have access to warm, nurturing relationships with loving caregivers, high-quality early childhood experiences, and ongoing monitoring of their developmental trajectories. Similarly, our concept of system building must encompass all sectors that influence families' capacity and well-being. We must broaden our efforts beyond child health, early care and education, and family support to engage such sectors as child welfare, housing, food and nutrition, neighborhood health and safety, transportation, economic development, workforce deployment, and employment. Such cross-sector collaboration is essential to achieving our goal of supporting the developmental flourishing of all children through system transformation.

REFERENCES

1. American Academy of Pediatrics, Committee on Standards of Child Health Care. Standards of child health care. 2nd edition. Evanston (IL): American Academy of Pediatrics; 1972.
2. Hertzman C. Putting the concept of biological embedding in historical perspective. Proc Natl Acad Sci U S A 2012;109(Suppl 2):17160–7.
3. National Research Council and Institute of Medicine, Committee on Integrating the Science of Early Childhood Development, Shonkoff JP, et al, editors. Board on Children, Youth, and Families, Commission on Behavioral and Social Sciences and Education. From neurons to neighborhoods: the science of early childhood development. Washington, DC: National Academy Press; 2000.
4. Navsaria D, editor. Early brain and child development. Building brains, forging futures. American Academy of Pediatrics. Available at: http://www.aap.org/en-us/advocacy-and-policy/aap-health-initiatives/EBCD/Pages/default.aspx. Accessed September 25, 2015.
5. Halfon N, Hochstein M. Life course health development: an integrated framework for developing health, policy, and research. Milbank Q 2002;80(3):433–79.
6. Chamberlin RW. Preventing low birth weight, child abuse, and school failure: the need for comprehensive, community-wide approaches. Pediatr Rev 1992;13(2): 64–71.
7. World Health Organization. Commission on Social Determinants of Health. 2004. Available at: http://apps.who.int/iris/bitstream/10665/20230/1/B115_35-en.pdf. Accessed October 3, 2015.
8. McGinnis JM, Williams-Russo P, Knickman JR. The case for more active policy attention to health promotion. Health Aff 2002;21(2):78–93.
9. National Center for Health Statistics. Percentage of children with serious emotional or behavioral difficulties, by age group and family income group—National Health Interview Survey, United States, 2004–2009. MMWR Morb Mortal Wkly Rep 2011;60(17):555.
10. Child Health Advocacy Committee. Workgroup on the role of children's hospitals in health and wellness. Washington, DC: Children's Hospital Association: Creating Health; 2014.
11. Taylor C. Cost-benefit of "demedicalizing" childhood developmental and behavioral concerns: national replication of *Help Me Grow*. 2012. Available at: http://www.helpmegrownational.org/includes/research/PolicyBrief_FINAL_31MAY2012.pdf. Accessed September 25, 2015.
12. American Academy of Pediatrics, Council on Children With Disabilities, Section on Developmental Behavioral Pediatrics, Bright Futures Steering Committee, Medical Home Initiatives for Children With Special Needs Project Advisory Committee. Identifying infants and young children with developmental disorders in the medical home: an algorithm for developmental surveillance and screening. Pediatrics 2006;118:405–20.
13. Dworkin PH. Historical overview: from ChildServ to *Help Me Grow*. J Dev Behav Pediatr 2006;27:S5–7.

14. McKay KA, Vater S, Dworkin PH. ChildServ: lessons learned from the design and implementation of a community-based developmental surveillance program. Inf Young Child 2006;19:371–7.

15. Connecticut Department of Social Services, Department of Children and Families. Connecticut community KidCare status report. April 1, 2004 – June 30, 2004. Available at: http://www.ct.gov/dcf/LIB/dcf/behavioral_health/pdf/KidCare_Q4_04.pdf. Accessed October 3, 2015.

16. Connecticut State Department of Education. Results-based accountability. Available at: http://www.sde.ct.gov/sde/cwp/view.asp?a=2711&Q=322618. Accessed September 25, 2015.

17. Hughes M, Damboise MC. Help Me Grow: 2008 annual evaluation report. Available at: http://www.ct.gov/ctf/lib/ctf/HMG_Report_2007-2008.pdf. Accessed September 25, 2015.

18. Smith KB, Larimer CW. The public policy primer. Boulder (CO): Westview Press; 2009.

19. Center for the Study of Social Policy. The protective factors framework. Available at: http://www.cssp.org/reform/strengthening-families/basic-one-pagers/Strengthening-Families-Protective-Factors.pdf. Accessed September 25, 2015.

20. Hughes M, Joslyn A, Wojton M, et al. Connecting vulnerable children and families to community-based programs strengthens parents' perceptions of protective factors. Inf Young Child 2016, in press.

21. *Help Me Grow* National Center. Home page. Available at: http://www.helpmegrownational.org/. Accessed September 25, 2015.

22. Pillas D, Marmot M, Naicker K, et al. Social inequities in early childhood health and development: a European-wide systematic review. Pediatr Res 2014;76(5):418–24.

23. Garg A, Sandel M, Dworkin PH, et al. From medical home to health neighborhood: transforming the medical home into a community-based health neighborhood. J Pediatr 2013;160:535–6.

24. Children's Hospital Association. Optimizing health care for children with medical complexity. Available at: https://www.childrenshospitals.org/~/media/Files/CHA/Main/Issues_and_Advocacy/Key_Issues/Children_With_Medical_Complexity/Issue%20Briefs%20and%20Reports/OptimizingHealthCareReport_10152013.pdf. Accessed October 3, 2015.

25. Kavanagh J, Gerdes M, Sell K, et al. Series: an integrated approach to supporting child development. Philadelphia: Policy Lab, The Children's Hospital of Philadelphia Research Institute; 2012. Available at: http://policylab.chop.edu/sites/default/files/pdf/publications/PolicyLab_EtoA_SERIES_Developmental_Screening_Summer_2012.pdf. Accessed September 25, 2015.

Appendix

Ross A. Yaple, MD[a],*, Kerry O'Loughlin, BA[b,c], Jim Hudziak, MD[d]

KEYWORDS

- Mental health promotion • Access to health care • Child development
- Education programs • Violence prevention • Poverty reduction • Data registry
- Social system improvements

KEY POINTS

- Several programs have been developed that focus on mental and general health promotion and prevention strategies that aim to improve access to care and utilization of services for underserved populations.
- Evidence-based data registries are available that review the quality of social programs and identify promising and model strategies and initiatives for health promotion.
- Currently, many innovative interventions have demonstrated improvements in areas of social capital, such as abuse and violence prevention; poverty reduction; maternal health; child development; obesity reduction; academic success; and community enhancements.

INTRODUCTION

This article is designed to serve as a reference for researchers and clinicians interested in extant evidence-based programs designed to promote healthy youth development. As such, this article begins with a review of 2 freely available online registries of evidence-based youth development programs. Both registries compile information on healthy youth development programs and rate such programs on pre-established criteria. The 2 registries outlined here are

- Blueprints for Healthy Youth Development
- The Social Research Unit

Conflicts of Interest: None.
[a] Division of Child and Adolescent Psychiatry, Virginia Treatment Center for Children, Children's Hospital of Richmond, Virginia Commonwealth University Health System, 515 North 10th Street, Richmond, VA 23298, USA; [b] Department of Psychological Science, The Unversity of Vermont, Dewey Hall, Rm 248, 2 Colchester Avenue, Burlington, VT 05401, USA; [c] Department of Psychiatry, The University of Vermont College of Medicine, The University Health Center Campus, St. Joseph's Wing, 1 South Prospect Street, Burlington, VT 05401, USA; [d] Fletcher Allen Health Care, University of Vermont College of Medicine, 1 South Prospect Street, Burlington, VT 05495, USA
* Corresponding author.
E-mail address: ross.yaple@vcuhealth.org

Child Adolesc Psychiatric Clin N Am 25 (2016) 319–335
http://dx.doi.org/10.1016/j.chc.2015.11.010
1056-4993/16/$ – see front matter © 2016 Elsevier Inc. All rights reserved.

childpsych.theclinics.com

This article also outlines several specific model programs, which intervene on a variety of targets to promote healthy youth development. The model programs described here are

- Social Development Research Group
- Nurse-Family Partnership
- Gatehouse Project
- Magnolia Place Community Initiative (MPCI)
- Harlem Children's Zone (HCZ)
- Conditional cash transfer (CCT)
- Live Well San Diego/Healthy Works
- Help Me Grow National Center (HMG)

Lastly, this article outlines emerging youth development programs, namely

- Synchrony Project (SP)
- Harmony Project (HP)
- Vermont Family Based Approach (VFBA)

The model and emerging programs reviewed in this article have resulted in myriad positive outcomes, which include enhancing community engagement, promoting healthy choices, facilitating access to resources, improving academic engagement, improving academic achievement, promoting prenatal health, and fostering social-emotional development. The authors hope this article serves as a useful resource for those interested in evidence-based strategies to promote healthy youth development as well as a source of inspiration for future work.

BLUEPRINTS FOR HEALTHY YOUTH DEVELOPMENT

The Blueprints for Healthy Youth Development provides "a registry of evidence-based youth development programs designed to promote the health and well being of children and teens."[1] The Blueprints program began in 1996 with funding from the State of Colorado and the US Department of Justice Office of Juvenile Justice and Delinquency Prevention and was designed to prevent youth violence, crime, and drug use.[2] Currently, Blueprints focuses on a variety of outcomes relating to positive youth development and is funded by the Annie E. Casey Foundation. The Blueprints program was initiated at and continues to be housed at the Center for the Study and Prevention of Violence (CSPV) at the Institute of Behavioral Science, University of Colorado Boulder.[1]

The goals of the Blueprints initiative are 4-fold:

- Identify effective, research-based programs
- Provide training and technical assistance to transfer the requisite knowledge and skills to implement these programs
- Monitor the implementation process to provide feedback to sites and ensure that programs are implemented with fidelity to their original intent and design
- Gather and disseminate information regarding factors that enhance the quality and fidelity of implementation[3]

The Blueprints program has developed and implemented research-based criteria for evaluating program effectiveness. In the Blueprints model, program effectiveness is based on an initial review by CSPV and a final review and recommendation from an advisory board, currently comprised of 7 experts in the field of positive youth development. This review process results in the identification of programs that have been effective in reducing problem behaviors and promoting healthy youth development. Such programs are identified as "promising," "model," or "model plus," and such programs serve as Blueprints.[4]

Per the Blueprints evaluation process, for a program to be denoted as promising, model, or model plus, the following standards must be met.

Promising programs evidence

1. Intervention specificity: "The program description clearly identifies the outcome the program is designed to change, the specific risk and/or protective factors targeted to produce this change in outcome, the population for which it is intended, and how the components of the intervention work to produce this change."
2. Evaluation quality: "The evaluation trials produce valid and reliable findings. This requires a minimum of (a) one high quality randomized control trial or (b) two high quality quasi-experimental evaluations."
3. Intervention impact: "The evidence from the high quality evaluations indicates significant positive change in intended outcomes that can be attributed to the program and there is no evidence of harmful effects."
4. Dissemination readiness: "The program is currently available for dissemination and has the necessary organizational capability, manuals, training, technical assistance and other support required for implementation with fidelity in communities and public service systems."

Model programs meet these additional standards

5. Evaluation quality: "A minimum of (a) two high quality randomized control trials or (b) one high quality randomized control trial plus one high quality quasi-experimental evaluation."
6. Positive intervention impact is "sustained for a minimum of 12 months after the program intervention ends."

Finally, model plus programs meet 1 additional standard

7. Independent replication: "In at least one high quality study demonstrating desired outcomes, authorship, data collection, and analysis has been conducted by a researcher who is neither a current or past member of the program developer's research team and who has no financial interest in the program."[4]

To date, the Blueprints program has reviewed more than 1300 programs and less than 5% have been identified as promising or model, and the CSPV continues to review programs that meet the selection criteria.[1] To date, the following programs have met the model or model plus program selection criteria: Blues Program (Cognitive Behavioral Group Depression Prevention), Body Project (dissonance intervention), Brief Alcohol Screening and Intervention for College Students, Functional Family Therapy, LifeSkills Training, Multisystemic Therapy for Youth with Problem Sexual Behaviors, Multisystemic Therapy, New Beginnings (intervention for children of divorce), Nurse-Family Partnership, Parent Management Training (Oregon Model), Project Towards No Drug Abuse (Positive Action), Promoting Alternative Thinking Strategies, and Treatment Foster Care Oregon.[5]

When funding has been available, the Blueprints initiative has also provided communities with technical assistance and monitoring so that communities can plan for and develop effective interventions. The Office of Juvenile Justice and Delinquency Prevention funded replications of Blueprints programs nationwide—"delivering training and technical assistance to 42 sites replicating 8 of the Blueprints model violence prevention programs and implementing a model drug prevention program to another 105 sites (representing approximately 400 schools)."[3]

THE SOCIAL RESEARCH UNIT

Royston Lambert founded the Social Research Unit in 1963 at King's College Cambridge. It was initially designed to examine how children's services influenced the well-being of children from underprivileged backgrounds. In 1968, the Social Research Unit became part of the Dartington Hall Trust and in 2003 became an independent charity.[6]

Currently, the Social Research Unit is based in Dartington, United Kingdom, and remains an independent charity focused on "generating the data and evidence that decision-makers need in order to make informed decisions that will improve children's outcomes across the education, health, social care and criminal justice systems."[7] The Social Research Unit evaluates programs based on the following foci:

1. Intervention specificity – "is the intervention focused, practical, logical and designed based on the best available evidence?"
2. Evaluation quality – "is the evaluation design and execution robust enough to permit confidence in the results?"
3. Intervention impact – "what do robust evaluations tell us about how much impact the intervention has on key developmental outcomes for children?"
4. System readiness – "can the intervention be implemented in the 'real world' context of a public service system?"[8]

Using these standards, the Social Research Unit has developed a registry of programs, freely available online. The registry indicates the program's cost-benefit ratio, return on investment, risk of loss, and whether the program met the Blueprints for Healthy Youth Development standards. The Social Research Unit relies on a method of cost-benefit analysis developed in the United States by the Washington State Institute for Public Policy.[9]

In an effort to implement early intervention strategies designed to improve child outcomes and produce financial savings, the Social Research Unit, using its Evidence2-Success method, has collaborated with local authorities in communities, such as Birmingham (England), Perth and Kinross (Scotland), and Providence, Rhode Island (United States). During these collaborations, the Social Research Unit provides data on children's needs and cost-benefit analyses at the local level. Such information is then used to delineate how existing funds are spent on children, inform evidence-based commissioning strategies, and promote shifts in spending toward evidence-based prevention and early intervention.[10]

SOCIAL DEVELOPMENT RESEARCH GROUP

Based at the University of Washington School of Social Work, the Social Development Research Group is an interdisciplinary group of researchers who aim to understand and promote healthy behaviors and positive social development. The goals of the group are to (1) conduct research on factors that influence development, (2) develop and test the effectiveness of interventions, (3) study service systems and work to improve them, (4) advocate for science-based solutions to health and behavior problems, and (5) disseminate knowledge, tools, and expertise generated by the Social Development Research Group.[11]

Notable among the myriad studies conducted by the Social Development Research Group is the Community Youth Development Study. The Community Youth

Development Study began in 2003 and is a community-based randomized trial of the effectiveness of the Communities That Care (CTC) prevention system. The CTC prevention system is designed to promote healthy youth development and reduce levels of youth drug use, violence, delinquency, teenage pregnancy, and school dropout.[12] Broadly, CTC empowers communities to collect and use community-specific data on risk and protective factors and to use that data to guide the selection of prevention programs tailored to a community's specific needs.[12] Installation of CTC includes completion of 5 phases:

1. Get started—assessing community readiness to undertake collaborative prevention efforts
2. Get organized—getting a commitment to the CTC process from community leaders and forming a diverse and representative prevention coalition
3. Develop a profile—using epidemiologic data to assess prevention needs and evaluating gaps in current services related to those needs
4. Create a plan—choosing tested and effective prevention policies, practices, and programs based on assessment data
5. Implement and evaluate—implementing the new policies, programs, and practices with fidelity, in a manner congruent with the program's theory, content, and methods of delivery, and evaluating progress over time[12]

The CTC prevention system was tested in 24 communities across 7 states, with these communities randomly assigned to receive the CTC intervention or to serve as controls.[13] Research suggests that children in CTC communities are less likely than children in control communities to use drugs, drink alcohol, smoke cigarettes, engage in delinquent behavior, and commit violent acts.[14] Such positive effects seem long lasting, with research suggesting that 15 years after the CTC intervention, children involved in CTC communities had significantly better educational and economic attainment, mental health, and sexual health by age 27.[15]

THE NURSE-FAMILY PARTNERSHIP

The Nurse-Family Partnership program is a nonprofit maternal health program, which provides high-risk, first-time parents with maternal and child health nurses.[16] In the United States, The Nurse-Family Partnership is utilized in 43 states and the US Virgin Islands.[17] The aim of The Nurse-Family Partnership is to provide first-time mothers with skills and support so that they can have healthy pregnancies, gain knowledge about parenting, and become responsible parents.[16]

Three randomized controlled trials (Elmira, New York, 1977; Memphis, Tennessee, 1990; and Denver, Colorado, 1994) examined the efficacy of the Nurse-Family Partnership program.[18] Each of these trials enrolled first-time, low-income mothers and follow-up research is ongoing. Positive effects demonstrated in at least 2 of the 3 randomized controlled trials include improved prenatal health, fewer childhood injuries, fewer closely spaced subsequent pregnancies, increased intervals between births, increased maternal employment, improved school readiness, reductions in use of welfare and other government assistance, greater maternal employment, and greater partner stability.[18]

The Nurse Family Partnership has also demonstrated reductions in child abuse and neglect, as well as reductions in number of trips to the emergency department during a child's second year of life.[19,20] Families involved with The Nurse-Family Partnership program also showed evidence of reductions in health care encounters for child injuries and ingestions as well as reductions in the number of days that children spent hospitalized with injuries and ingestions during the first 2 years of life.[21]

The Nurse-Family Partnership also seems to mitigate the impact of maternal psychopathology on child outcomes. In the Memphis trial, nurse-visited children born to mothers with higher levels of depression and anxiety and lower levels of intellectual functioning and sense of mastery over their lives had better academic achievement compared with their counterparts in the control group. Similarly, in the Denver trial, nurse-visited 4 year olds born to mothers with higher levels of depression, anxiety and lower levels of intellectual functioning and sense of mastery over their lives evidenced better language development and greater impulse control than children in the control group.[22]

THE GATEHOUSE PROJECT

The Gatehouse Project was a research project conducted in Victoria, Australia, secondary schools between 1996 and 2001. The Gatehouse Project was funded by the Queen's Trust for Young Australians (subsequently Foundation for Young Australians), the Victorian Health Promotion Foundation (VicHealth), the National Health and Medical Research Council (Australia), the Department of Human Services (Victoria, Australia), the Sidney Myer Foundation, and the Baker Foundation.[23]

The Gatehouse Project framework conceptualizes the promotion of students' mental health as a school's responsibility and relies on a framework in which students' emotional-behavioral health is seen as a function of each child's sense of positive connection with teachers, peers, and learning. The Gatehouse Project has identified 3 priority areas for action:

1. "Building a sense of security and trust"
2. "Enhancing skills and opportunities for communication and social connectedness"
3. "Building a sense of positive regard through valued participation in school life"[24]

The Gatehouse Project program is designed to start when students are 13 to 14 years of age and to continue for 2 years. The teachers at schools enrolled in the Gatehouse program receive approximately 40 hours of professional development, and the primary aims of the program are to increase levels of emotional well-being and to reduce rates of substance use and abuse.[25]

A randomized controlled trial of the Gatehouse Project, involving 26 schools and 2678 students, was conducted in Victoria, Australia. Schools were randomly assigned to either the Gatehouse intervention or the control group. Data were collected from students at the beginning of 8th grade and at the end of 8th, 9th, and 10th grades. Results suggest that relative to the control group, students involved in the Gatehouse intervention reported personal reductions in drinking and smoking as well as reductions in the rate of alcohol and tobacco use among their friend group.[26]

THE MAGNOLIA PLACE COMMUNITY INITIATIVE – LOS ANGELES, CALIFORNIA

The MPCI is a collective of more than 70 government and community agencies that began in 2001 as a strategic planning process by the Children's Bureau of Southern California. Officially launched in 2008, the MPCI combines efforts through the community, city, and county to serve more than 35,000 children in 500 blocks in the Magnolia catchment area in Los Angeles.[27] The mission of the MPCI is to create safe, supportive environments for children and to reduce the burden of poverty, abuse, and neglect by strengthening individual, family, and community protective factors (**Boxes 1** and **2**).[28]

The MPCI strategy utilizes a "theory of community change" model that goes beyond traditional service delivery paradigms and emphasizes relationship-based organization between community residents. Neighborhood ambassadors and parent

---

Box 1
Magnolia Place Community Initiative's 4 core areas of development

- Educational success
- Economic stability
- Good health
- Safe and nurturing parenting

Data from Magnoliaplacela.org. Magnolia place. Available at: http://www.magnoliaplacela. org. Accessed August 2, 2015.

---

volunteers engage with residents in the community to form action groups, who then contribute to improvements in social capital through community transformation projects, support groups, and policy change.[27]

The MPCI tracks progress toward major goals through monthly surveys that form the community data dashboard, with specific focus in the following areas:

- Vulnerability versus readiness for kindergarten
- Reading proficiency
- Parents of children with protective factors and achievement of family goals
- Parents reading with children
- Social ties to neighbors
- Assistance with financial stressors
- Parents asked about depression
- Parent discussions about family resources, development concerns, and family stressors

Ultimately, the goal of the MPCI is scalable and sustainable community-level change, where all of the children and families in the catchment area achieve success in education, health, economic stability and quality, and nurturing care.[29]

THE HARLEM CHILDREN'S ZONE—NEW YORK, NEW YORK

The HCZ is a nonprofit organization that began in the 1990s as a single-block community redevelopment project in central Harlem. After a 10-year strategic plan in 2000,

---

Box 2
Magnolia Place Community Initiative's 6 protective factors

- Parental resilience
- Knowledge of parenting
- Social and emotional development
- Nurturing and attachment
- Social connections
- Concrete support in times of need

Data from Bowie P. Getting to scale: the elusive goal. Seattle (WA): Casey Family Programs; 2011. Available at: http://www.magnoliaplacela.org/resources/GettingToScale_MagnoliaPlace. pdf. Accessed August 2, 2015.

---

the program has expanded to serve more than 13,000 youth as well as 13,000 adults across 97 blocks in Harlem.[30]

The vision of the HCZ is to have all children living in the catchment area break the multigenerational cycle of poverty by successfully graduating from college and becoming self-sustaining adults. The HCZ works to achieve these goals through large-scale investments in educational programming, community redevelopment, and health initiatives.[30]

The HCZ educational initiatives began in 2000 with a focus on fostering child development and parenting workshops and expanded to include preschool programs, charter schools, and college preparation as well as counseling services for those graduates who have entered college (**Box 3**). The HCZ reports a 92% college acceptance rate across all of its programs as well as achievement scores that have surpassed public school systems across New York State. In addition to classroom learning, the HCZ offers its students counseling services, on-site nutrition, medical and dental services, tutoring, parent workshops, and financial literacy as well as employment and technology services to enhance occupational skills.[30]

Independent review by the Harvard University Department of Economics in 2011 reported that the HCZ program successfully closed the racial achievement gap in both mathematics and English for elementary school students and for mathematics in middle school.[31,32]

In addition to educational initiatives, the HCZ has also created community development programs to improve social connection and safe spaces to learn and develop (**Box 4**).[30] Programs, such as the Beacon Community Centers and Community Pride, work with local tenants, associations, and businesses to revitalize the community and provide employment workshops, legal assistance, and tax preparation. Health initiatives, such as Healthy Harlem and the Asthma Initiative, focus on nutrition, fitness activities, and health outcomes for children and families.[30,33]

CONDITIONAL CASH TRANSFER

CCT programs are systems that distribute cash incentives to poor households with the expectation that the household will engage in specified investments in the welfare of their children.[34] In most cases, the specified investments include health and educational measures, such as

- Annual physician visits and health checkups
- Growth monitoring
- Vaccinations
- Perinatal care

Box 3
Harlem Children's Zone's education programs

- Early development: Baby College, Baby College GRADS, and Three-Year-Old Journey
- Preschool program: Harlem Gems
- Promise Academy Charter Schools
- College Preparatory Program
- College Success Office

Data from Harlem Children's Zone. Home - harlem children's zone. 2015. Available at: http://www.hcz.org. Accessed August 2, 2015.

Box 4
Harlem Children's Zone's community and health programs

- HCZ community centers
- Beacon Community Centers
- Foster care prevention program
- Single Stop and Tax Preparation Program
- Healthy Harlem
- Harlem Armory
- Safety Knights

Data from Harlem Children's Zone. Home - harlem children's zone. 2015. Available at: http://www.hcz.org. Accessed August 2, 2015.

- School enrollment
- School attendance

CCT programs have demonstrated significant expansion since 1997, especially in underdeveloped countries. Nearly every country in Latin America utilizes some form of CCT, with expanding presence in Asia, Southeast Asia, and Africa. Many of these countries have implemented CCT as part of larger government social protection systems with the aim of direct reduction in poverty rates and redistribution of capital. Outcomes have largely been mixed, with improvements in utilization of health services and increased school enrollment offset by limited gains in actual health or educational outcomes, although programs with very early intervention incentives may demonstrate improvements in cognitive development.[34]

The first comprehensive CCT program in a developed country was the Opportunity NYC–Family Rewards program established in 2007 by the NYC Center for Economic Opportunity.[35] The program covered 4800 families and 11,000 children in the 6 poorest areas in New York City until the project closed in 2010. The program was privately funded and set up as a randomized controlled trial with half of the families eligible for cash incentive rewards. The Family Rewards program was successful in the reduction of current poverty and material hardship, hunger, and increasing family savings, although the gains diminished once the program ended. There were no significant educational gains in terms of outcomes, except for improved graduation rates for high school students who entered high school as proficient readers. Health outcomes were limited to increases in use of preventive dental measures, because utilization of preventive health services was already high in the population studied. The Opportunity NYC–Family Rewards model is currently being reconfigured and studied in Bronx, New York, and in Memphis, Tennessee.[35]

LIVE WELL SAN DIEGO/HEALTHY WORKS—SAN DIEGO, CALIFORNIA

The Live Well San Diego/Healthy Works program is a county-wide health initiative designed to reduce tobacco use, poor nutrition, and physical inactivity, the 3 leading risk factors for heart and lung disease, cancer, and diabetes for residents in the area. Launched in 2010 through the County of San Diego Health and Human Services Agency in collaboration with the Centers for Disease Control and Prevention, the program engages local residents, schools, businesses, and policy makers with the goal of improving access to healthy food choices through global nutrition education as well as improving activity levels through city planning and development.[36,37]

The Healthy Works nutrition agenda includes programs that support sustainable community food production, access to fresh fruits and vegetables in retail stores as well as in school meal programs, and interactive nutrition classes for families as well as marketing programs to raise awareness of locally grown, certified foods (**Box 5**). Physical activity programs include city development projects, such as Complete Streets to create safe roads for cyclists and pedestrians to share with vehicle traffic, and obesity prevention programs in schools and physical activity breaks in the workplace and communities. Smoke-free policies were instituted in all multiunit housing and apartments in 2013. Healthy Works also introduced resident-led community impact programs focused on creating communities of excellence and increasing awareness on nutrition and obesity prevention as well as quality-of-life initiatives, including health impact assessments for land use and transportation planning projects.[37]

THE HELP ME GROW NATIONAL CENTER—HARTFORD, CONNECTICUT

The HMG program is an innovative model that connects families and clinicians to area services with a focus on early identification of developmental and behavioral problems in children from birth to 8 years old.[38] Originally started as ChildServ in 1998 through

---

Box 5
Healthy Works programs

Healthy eating
- Community Agriculture Planning Project
- Healthy retail
- Healthy school meals
- Nutrition education
- San Diego Grown 365
- Workplace lactation

Active living
- Complete Streets
- Increasing physical activity in schools
- Instant Fitness
- Successful safe routes to schools

Tobacco-free living
- Live Well @ Work
- Smoke-free multiunit housing

Healthy communities
- Communities of Excellence
- Faith-Based Wellness
- Health impact assessment
- Healthy Communities Campaign
- Resident Leadership Academy

Data from Healthyworks.org. Paths to healthy living | healthy works. Available at: http://www.healthyworks.org. Accessed August 2, 2015.

the University of Connecticut Medical Center in conjunction with state government agencies and the United Way, HMG was initially replicated in Orange County in 2005 and since has expanded to have affiliate programs in 23 states.[39]

The HMG National Center program uses 4 core components (**Box 6**) in a simplistic model that emphasizes a single point of entry and centralized assistance in navigating complex health resource systems. HMG staff travel to areas of affiliate programs and provide training in developmental and behavioral screening to clinicians and also meet with community agencies to provide networking and coordination among services to maximize patient access through the maintenance of a resource directory. The Child Development Infoline serves as the access center for families and clinicians with questions or to make a referral, and the call center staff also provide education to the families, including mailing stage–based developmental screens that families can complete with their children.[40]

Data on the HMG program demonstrate that 85% of families called are successfully referred to appropriate services.[38] A survey of families served by HMG in 2012 demonstrated positive effects in building resiliency in families and optimizing child development, improved family knowledge of development and access to services, and improvements in parent-child relationships, child behavior, and parenting practices.[41]

THE SYNCHRONY PROJECT—ST LOUIS, MISSOURI

The SP is a collaboration between Washington University in St. Louis, the St Louis County Family Court, and the Children's Division of the Missouri Department of Social Services that provides in-depth family assessments targeting youth most at risk for abuse and neglect: 0 to 5 year olds within the foster care system. Funded by the Children's Service Fund of St Louis County, the SP aims to provide preventive supports and interventions to reduce the overall risk burden as early as possible in the developmental course of the children and families served.[42]

Developed from previous evidence on intervention programs for maltreated infants[43] and adverse outcomes for those with additive risk factors,[44] the SP provides intensive evaluations of children with identified histories of abuse and neglect, along with their foster parents and biological parents, by a team of psychiatrists, psychologists, social workers, and family court representatives. The sessions include multiple direct observations of the parent/child relationship, including standardized assessments of child and caregiver engagement, affect, direction, responsivity, and disciplinary control, with the goal of creating a system of interventions to best assist each family. The SP model utilizes a strengths-based approach with the ultimate goal of family reunification when possible, and recommendations are made to the family court with follow-up plans that have the primary focus of intergenerational mental

---

Box 6
Help Me Grow National Center's core components

- Physician outreach

- Community outreach

- Centralized call center

- Data collection

Data from Helpmegrownational.org. Help Me Grow National Center. Available at: http://www. helpmegrownational.org. Accessed August 2, 2015.

health care delivery as well as an evidence-based group parenting education program developed at Washington University.[42]

Data from the SP demonstrated that 85% of families referred to the program participate in the interventions and that a significant proportion of these families had not engaged in medically indicated interventions, including evidence-based therapies for developmental delay or untreated mental illness, at the time of the initial assessment. Additional data indicate significant differences on the impact of detection of families with a prior history of adjudication as well as changes in court dispositions and reunification rates to abusive families.[45]

THE HARMONY PROJECT—LOS ANGELES, CALIFORNIA

The HP is a nonprofit organization that provides music instruction and ensemble performance experiences for low-income youth. Founded in 2001 in Los Angeles through funding from the Rotary Club of Hollywood, the HP has since expanded to 17 sites in Los Angeles as well as programs in 7 other major cities across the United States and has served thousands of children. The HP was founded on the premise that engaging at-risk youth in the arts and music can reduce the impact of gangs in some of the most violent areas by improving the sense of community through music education. The mission of the HP focuses on 3 main areas (**Box 7**).[46]

The HP has been successful in establishing several youth-based projects in Los Angeles, including the Youth Orchestra Los Angeles, chamber orchestras, and a Hip Hop Orchestra. Students receive several hours of musical instruction per week, and private funding has allowed for youth from low-income backgrounds to receive high-quality instruments free of charge. A peer mentorship program was established in 2010, which allows advanced students to teach younger students in exchange for professional private lessons. Students who develop excellence in talent and a desire for a career in music benefit from the Academy at HP, which provides additional training opportunities per week. Many students have received educational scholarships through the HP program.[46]

The HP uses a research-based model and partnered with the Northwestern University Auditory Neurosciences Laboratory in 2013, resulting in several studies that have demonstrated significant gains in neural auditory processing mechanisms linked with reading and language skills.[47,48] Recent impact surveys of the HP have also demonstrated parent-rated improvements in mood, health, grades, and behaviors as well as significant impacts in high school graduation rates and college attendance compared with low-income youth in high crime areas of Los Angeles who do not participate in HP.[46]

Box 7
The Harmony Project's mission

- The promotion of growth and development through the study, practice, and performance of music

- To build healthier communities by investing in the positive development of children through music

- To develop children as musical ambassadors of peace, hope, and understanding amongst people of diverse cultures, backgrounds, and beliefs

Data from Harmony-project.org. Harmony project. 2015. Available at: http://www.harmony-project.org. Accessed September 5, 2015.

THE VERMONT FAMILY BASED APPROACH

The VFBA is a clinical and public health paradigm based on the following foci: (1) emotional-behavioral health is the cornerstone of all health; (2) health is familial; and (3) health promotion, prevention, and intervention are essential for enhancing population health. The VFBA was developed by Dr Jim Hudziak, Director of the Vermont Center for Children, Youth, and Families at the University of Vermont Medical Center.[49]

The VFBA is designed to integrate extant research on developmental psychopathology into a family-based therapeutic intervention. The VFBA hinges on the notion that if either parent in a family suffers from psychopathology, then the children in that family are at increased risk for psychopathology.[50–52] Research indicates that environment contributes as much to risk as genes,[53,54] and the VFBA is designed to improve the milieu in which a child lives by treating not only a child's emotional-behavioral illness but also his or her parents' emotional-behavioral struggles.

Therapeutically, The VFBA relies on a therapeutic model in which a family wellness coach, a focused family coach, and a family-based psychiatrist treat a child's entire family. The family wellness coach provides a comprehensive program of coaching on health and wellness to the whole family, including nutrition, exercise, healthy activities, music training, reading programs, sports programs, peer support program, physical and mental health, and effective parenting. The focused family coach delivers evidence-based psychotherapeutic interventions from the family perspective, and the family-based psychiatrist delivers evidence-based psychotherapeutic and psychopharmacologic interventions from the family perspective. The VFBA is based on the notion that a child's emotional-behavioral well-being is intimately related to the family environment.

Components of the VFBA have also been translated into school-based settings. Elements of the VFBA have been implemented in school-based programs in Garfield, South Dakota, and the Mary Hogan School in Vermont.[55] In these programs, during the school day, health promotion is carried out in the form of instruction in Tai Chi, violin, and sports, with prevention and intervention relying on evidence-based treatments of parents and children.[55] Several grants have also sought to examine the underlying tenants of the VFBA, including the National Healthcare Group (NHG)-Singapore SIG 1 grant (primary investigator: Sharon Cohan Sung, PhD), as well as the ZonMw 40-00812-98-10020 grant in the Netherlands (primary investigator: Christine Middeldorp, MD, PhD).[55]

A randomized clinical trial of the Family Assessment and Feedback Intervention (FAFI), a component of the VFBA, began in the fall of 2015. This randomized clinical trial is funded by the Bi-State Primary Care Association and is being conducted at the Health Center (Plainfield, Vermont), a Federally Qualified Health Center. The FAFI is a brief, manualized, family-focused intervention that uses evidence-based assessment with feedback in a motivational enhancement framework. The FAFI involves engaging family members in a discussion of the "results of assessment of both children's and parents' competencies and problems and the family environment using Motivational Interviewing techniques." Ultimately FAFI is designed to enhance parents' and children's treatment engagement with mental health services to ultimately improve children's clinical outcomes.[56]

A randomized clinical trial of the VFBA commenced in the fall of 2015. This trial is projected to include 120 to 160 families with a child between the ages of 3 to 6, and is being conducted at the University of Vermont Medical Center. The experimental group in this trial will include 60 to 80 families, and these families will be partnered with a family wellness coach, who will help them implement an individualized plan of family health and wellness based on the results of their family-based assessment. The plan will address the following aspects of family health and well-being using evidence-based health promotion and prevention strategies: nutrition, exercise, music, mindfulness, and positive parenting. Family wellness coaches will also work with families to overcome significant challenges of living, such as food, housing, and vocational insecurity. Families with a member experiencing significant emotional and behavioral problems will also be partnered with a focused family coach (a family-based, evidence-based psychotherapist) and a family-based psychiatrist. Children will be offered 30-minute group music lessons for the duration of the study. Each child will be invited to take part in up to 4 such lessons per week. While children attend music lessons, parents will be offered classes in a variety of healthy activities, including positive parenting, nutrition, cooking, and relaxation techniques. The control group will include 60 to 80 families and receive the assessment protocol along with financial remuneration. Results of this trial are forthcoming.

REFERENCES

1. Blueprintsprograms.com. Blueprints for healthy youth development. 2012-2015. Available at: http://www.blueprintsprograms.com/about.php. Accessed August 30, 2015.
2. Center for the Study and Prevention of Violence Institute of Behavioral Science University of Colorado Boulder. Blueprints background. Available at: http://www.colorado.edu/cspv/blueprints/background.html. Accessed August 30, 2015.
3. Mihalic S, Fagan A, Irwin K, et al. Blueprints for violence prevention. Report by Office of Juvenile Justice and Prevention. 2004. Available at: https://www.ncjrs.gov/pdffiles1/ojjdp/204274.pdf. Accessed August 30, 2015.
4. Blueprintsprograms.com. Blueprints for healthy youth development program criteria. 2012-2015. Available at: http://www.blueprintsprograms.com/program Criteria.php. Accessed August 30, 2015.
5. Blueprintsprograms.com. Blueprints for healthy youth development all programs. 2012-2015. Available at: http://www.blueprintsprograms.com/allPrograms.php. Accessed August 30, 2015.
6. King J. Dartington.org.uk. The social research unit about. 2015. Available at: http://dartington.org.uk/about/our-history/. Accessed August 30, 2015.
7. King J. Dartington.org.uk. The social research unit our work. 2015. Available at: http://dartington.org.uk/our-work/. Accessed August 30, 2015.
8. King J. Dartington.org.uk. The social research unit projects 'what works.' 2015. Available at: http://dartington.org.uk/projects/what-works-evidence-standards/. Accessed August 30, 2015.
9. King J. Dartington.org.uk. The Social Research Unit Projects Investing in Children. 2015. Available at: http://dartington.org.uk/projects/investing-in-children/. Accessed August 30, 2015.
10. King J. Dartington.org.uk. The social research unit projects evidence2success. 2015. Available at: http://dartington.org.uk/projects/evidence2success/. Accessed August 30, 2015.
11. Sdrg.org. Social development research group our mission. 2012. Available at: http://www.sdrg.org/mission.asp. Accessed August 30, 2015.
12. Communitiesthatcare.net. Communities that care how it works. 2015. Available at: http://www.communitiesthatcare.net/how-ctc-works/. Accessed August 30, 2015.
13. Communitiesthatcare.net. Communities that care research results. 2015. Available at: http://www.communitiesthatcare.net/research-results/. Accessed August 30, 2015.

14. Hawkins JD, Oesterle S, Brown EC, et al. Youth problem behaviors eight years after implementing the communities that care prevention system in a community-randomized trial. JAMA Pediatr 2014,168(2):122–9.
15. Hawkins JD, Kosterman R, Catalano RF, et al. Effects of social development intervention in childhood fifteen years later. Arch Pediatr Adolesc Med 2008;162(12):1133–41.
16. Nursefamilypartnership.org. Nurse family partnership home. 2011. Available at: http://www.nursefamilypartnership.org. Accessed August 30, 2015.
17. Nursefamilypartnership.org. Nurse family partnership fact sheet. 2015. Available at: http://www.nursefamilypartnership.org/assets/PDF/Factsheets/NFP_July_2015_Snapshot.aspx. Accessed August 30, 2015.
18. Nursefamilypartnership.org. Nurse family partnership proven results. 2015. Available at: http://www.nursefamilypartnership.org/proven-results. Accessed: August 30, 2015.
19. Olds D, Eckenrode J, Henderson C, et al. Long-term effects of home visitation on maternal life course and child abuse and neglect: a 15-year follow-up of a randomized trial. JAMA 1997;278(8):637–43.
20. Olds DL, Henderson CR Jr, Chamberlin R, et al. Preventing child abuse and neglect: a randomized trial of nurse home visitation. Pediatrics 1986;78(1):65–78.
21. Kitzman H, Olds DL, Henderson CR Jr, et al. Effect of prenatal and infancy home visitation by nurses on pregnancy outcomes, childhood injuries, and repeated childbearing: a randomized controlled trial. JAMA 1997;278(8):644–52.
22. Nursefamilypartnership.org. Nurse family partnership proven results improved school readiness. 2011. Available at: http://www.nursefamilypartnership.org/proven-results/Improve-school-readiness. Accessed August 30, 2015.
23. Rch.org.au. The royal children's hospital Melbourne the gatehouse project. Available at: http://www.rch.org.au/cah/research/The_Gatehouse_Project/. Accessed August 30, 2015.
24. Glover S, Patton G, Butler H, et al. The gatehouse project: promoting emotional well-being: team guidelines for whole school change. Victoria, Australia: Centre for Adolescent Health; 2002. Available at: http://www.mentalhealthpromotion.net/resources/gatehouse-project.pdf. Accessed August 30, 2015.
25. Childtrends.org. Child trends the gatehouse project. 2014. Available at: http://www.childtrends.org/?programs=the-gatehouse-project. Accessed August 30, 2015.
26. Bond L, Patton G, Glover S, et al. The gatehouse project: can a multilevel school intervention affect emotional wellbeing and health risk behaviours? J Epidemiol Community Health 2004;58(12):997–1003.
27. Magnoliaplacela.org. Magnolia place. Available at: http://www.magnoliaplacela.org. Accessed August 2, 2015.
28. Browne C. The strengthening families approach and protective factors framework: branching out and reaching deeper. Washington, DC: Center for the Study of Social Policy; 2014. Available at: http://www.cssp.org/reform/strengtheningfamilies/2014/The-Strengthening-Families-Approach-and-Protective-Factors-Framework_Branching-Out-and-Reaching-Deeper.pdf. Accessed August 2, 2015.
29. Bowie P. Getting to scale: the elusive goal. Seattle (WA): Casey Family Programs; 2011. Available at: http://www.magnoliaplacela.org/resources/GettingToScale_MagnoliaPlace.pdf. Accessed August 2, 2015.
30. Harlem Children's Zone. Home - Harlem children's zone. 2015. Available at: http://www.hcz.org. Accessed August 2, 2015.

31. Dobbie W, Fryer R. Are high-quality schools enough to increase achievement among the poor? Evidence from the Harlem children's zone. Am Econ J Appl Econ 2011;3(3):158–87.

32. Fryer R, Katz L. Achieving escape velocity: neighborhood and school interventions to reduce persistent inequality. Am Econ Rev 2013;103(3):232–7.

33. Nicholas S, Jean-Louis B, Ortiz B, et al. Addressing the childhood asthma crisis in Harlem: the Harlem children's zone asthma initiative. Am J Public Health 2005; 95(2):245–9.

34. Fiszbein A, Schady N. Conditional cash transfers. Washington, DC: World Bank; 2009.

35. Riccio J, DeChausay N, Miller C, et al. Conditional cash transfers in New York City: the continuing story of the opportunity-NYC – family rewards demonstration. 1st edition. New York: MDRC; 2013. Available at: http://www.mdrc.org/sites/default/files/Conditional_Cash_Transfers_FR_0.pdf. Accessed August 2, 2015.

36. Livewellsd.org. Home. Available at: http://www.livewellsd.org. Accessed August 2, 2015.

37. Healthyworks.org. Paths to healthy living | healthy works. Available at: http://www.healthyworks.org. Accessed August 2, 2015.

38. Helpmegrownational.org. Help Me Grow National Center. Available at: http://www.helpmegrownational.org. Accessed August 2, 2015.

39. Dworkin P. Historical overview. J Dev Behav Pediatr 2006;27(Supplement 1):S5–7.

40. Bogin J. Enhancing developmental services in primary care. J Dev Behav Pediatr 2006;27(Suppl 1):S8–12.

41. Hughes M, Joslyn A, Mora M, et al. Application of strengthening families framework to the help me grow model. Hartford (CT): Center for Social Research; 2012. Available at: http://ct.gov. Accessed August 2, 2015.

42. Doctor's Digest. SYNCHRONY project targets foster care's youngest at-risk children. 2011. Available at: http://www.stlouischildrens.org/sites/default/files/health_professionals/files/DocDigest_Aug11_web.pdf. Accessed September 5, 2015.

43. Jonson-Reid M, Presnall N, Drake B, et al. Effects of child maltreatment and inherited liability on antisocial development: an official records study. J Am Acad Child Adolesc Psychiatry 2010;49(4):321–32.

44. Zeanah C, Larrieu J, Heller S, et al. Evaluation of a preventive intervention for maltreated infants and toddlers in Foster care. J Am Acad Child Adolesc Psychiatry 2001;40(2):214–21.

45. Constantino J. The state of science and practice in the prevention of child abuse and neglect. Presented at the 2015 Midwest Justice for Children Conference. St. Charles (MO), April 1-3, 2015.

46. Harmony-project.org. Harmony project. 2015. Available at: http://www.harmony-project.org. Accessed September 5, 2015.

47. Kraus N, Hornickel J, Strait D, et al. Engagement in community music classes sparks neuroplasticity and language development in children from disadvantaged backgrounds. Front Psychol 2014;5:1403.

48. Kraus N, Slater J, Thompson E, et al. Music enrichment programs improve the neural encoding of speech in at-risk children. J Neurosci 2014;34(36):11913–8.

49. Hudziak JJ, Bartels M. Genetic and environmental influences on wellness, resilience, and psychopathology a family-based approach for promotion, prevention, and intervention. In: Hudziak JJ, editor. Developmental psychopathology and wellness. Arlington (VA): American Psychiatric Publishing Inc; 2008. p. 267–86.

50. Rijlaarsdam J, Stevens GW, Jansen PW, et al. Maternal childhood maltreatment and offspring emotional and behavioral problems: maternal and paternal mechanisms of risk transmission. Child Maltreat 2014;19(2):67–78.
51. Verhulst FC, Tiemeir H. Epidemiology of child psychopathology: major milestones. Eur Child Adolesc Psychiatry 2015;24(6):607–17.
52. Wadsworth ME, Rindlaub L, Hurwich-Reiss E, et al. A longitudinal examination of the adaptation to poverty-related stress model: predicting child and adolescent adjustment over time. J Clin Child Adolesc Psychol 2013;42(5):713–25.
53. Tiemeier H, Velders FP, Szekely E, et al. The generation R study: a review of design, findings to date, and a study of the 5-HTTLPR by environmental interaction from fetal life onward. J Am Acad Child Adolesc Psychiatry 2012;51(11): 1119–35.e7.
54. Boomsma DI, van Beijsterveldt CE, Hudziak JJ. Genetic and environmental influences on Anxious/Depression during childhood: a study from the Netherlands Twin Register. Genes Brain Behav 2005;4(8):466–81.
55. Hudziak, JJ. The Vemont family-based approach. 2010. Available at: https://www.uvm.edu/medicine/documents/CMS_Hudziak_Family_Approach_091410.pdf. Accessed September 8, 2015.
56. Vermont family-based approach. 2015. Available at: http://blog.uvm.edu/vfba/projects/. Accessed September 8, 2015.

Index

Note: Page numbers of article titles are in **boldface** type.

A

Abuse
    substance (*See* Substance abuse)
ACEs. *See* Adverse childhood experiences (ACEs)
ADHD. *See* Attention deficit hyperactivity disorder (ADHD)
Adolescence
    depression during
        prevention of, **201–218** (*See also* Depression, in childhood and adolescence,
            prevention of)
Adverse childhood experiences (ACEs)
    in ADHD, 140
    CDC/Kaiser Permanente study on, **139–156** (*See also* Centers for Disease Control and
        Prevention (CDC)/Kaiser Permanente study, on ACEs management)
    EMB disorders associated with, 140–141
    prevalence of, 140
    resilience and mindfulness-based approaches to, **139–156**
        discussion, 152–154
AOP. *See* Aussie Optimism Program (AOP)
Attention deficit hyperactivity disorder (ADHD)
    ACEs in, 140
Aussie Optimism Program (AOP)
    in depression prevention in childhood and adolescence, 208–209

B

Behavior(s)
    delinquent
        developmental course of, 258
    as precursors of severe delinquent behaviors, 258–259
Behavioral contracting
    in juvenile delinquency prevention, 261
Behavioral interventions
    in HIV prevention, 286–292
beyondblue
    in depression prevention in childhood and adolescence, 205
Biomedical interventions
    in HIV prevention, 286–292
Blueprints for Healthy Youth Development, 320–322
Brighter Futures initiative
    of HFPG, 311–312
Bully(ies)
    interventions for dealing with, 239

Child Adolesc Psychiatric Clin N Am 25 (2016) 337–348
http://dx.doi.org/10.1016/S1056-4993(16)30013-X
1056-4993/16/$ – see front matter © 2016 Elsevier Inc. All rights reserved.

Moving?

Make sure your subscription moves with you!

To notify us of your new address, find your **Clinics Account Number** (located on your mailing label above your name), and contact customer service at:

Email: **journalscustomerservice-usa@elsevier.com**

800-654-2452 (subscribers in the U.S. & Canada)
314-447-8871 (subscribers outside of the U.S. & Canada)

Fax number: **314-447-8029**

Elsevier Health Sciences Division
Subscription Customer Service
3251 Riverport Lane
Maryland Heights, MO 63043

*To ensure uninterrupted delivery of your subscription, please notify us at least 4 weeks in advance of move.

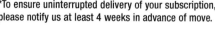
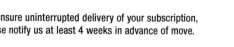